Principles of Hearing
Aid Audiology

Principles of Hearing Aid Audiology

Maryanne Tate

Springer-Science+Business Media, B.V.

First edition 1994

© Maryanne Tate 1994
Originally published by Maryanne Tate in 1994

ISBN 978-0-412-49070-5   ISBN 978-1-4899-7152-4 (eBook)
DOI 10.1007/978-1-4899-7152-4

A catalogue record for this book is available from the British Library

∞ Printed on permanent acid-free text paper, manufactured in
accordance with ANSI/NISO Z39.48-1992 and ANSI/NISO Z39.48-1984
(Permanence of Paper).

Contents

Foreword   ix
Acknowledgements   x

PART ONE   Fundamental Sciences   1

1 Acoustics   3
  1.1 Physical properties of sound   3
  1.2 The measurement of sound   10
  1.3 The audiometer   14
  1.4 The psychological properties of sound   17
  1.5 Summary   18
    References   19
    Further reading   19

2 Anatomy and physiology of the ear   20
  2.1 Anatomy of the ear   20
  2.2 The physiology of hearing   32
  2.3 Summary   39
    Further reading   40

3 Medical aspects of hearing loss   41
  3.1 Introduction   41
  3.2 Pathology of the outer ear   42
  3.3 Pathology of the middle ear   46
  3.4 Pathology of the inner ear   50
  3.5 Other conditions of the ear   57
  3.6 Summary   59
    References   60
    Further reading   60

4 Speech and intelligibility   61
  4.1 The speech chain   61

4.2 The vocal tract   63
4.3 Speech-reading   64
4.4 Speech sounds   65
4.5 Hearing loss and speech perception   70
4.6 Hearing loss and speech production   71
4.7 Summary   72
     Further reading   72

5 **The hearing aid system**   **73**
5.1 The basic components of a hearing aid   73
5.2 Elementary electricity and electronics   84
5.3 Signal processing   86
5.4 Summary   93
     References   94
     Further reading   94

PART TWO   **The Practice of Hearing Aid Audiology**   **95**

6 **The assessment procedure**   **97**
6.1 Pre-selection management   97
6.2 Otoscopy   101
6.3 Tuning fork tests   103
6.4 Principal audiometric tests   106
6.5 Understanding audiograms   117
6.6 Room requirements for audiometry   122
6.7 Summary   123
     References   124
     Further reading   125

7 **Hearing aids and their performance**   **126**
7.1 Introduction   126
7.2 Types of hearing aid system   127
7.3 Specification and performance   132
7.4 Hearing aid standards   139
7.5 Measuring methods   142
7.6 Power sources   146
7.7 The National Health Service provision of hearing aids 149
7.8 Summary   152
     References   153
     Further reading   153

8 **Selection and fitting**   **155**
8.1 The choice of a hearing aid system   155
8.2 Hearing aid fitting   163

8.3 Summary   171
    References   171
    Further reading   172

9 Earmoulds   173
9.1 Making the impression   173
9.2 Earmoulds   178
9.3 Summary   185
    References   185
    Further reading   186

10 Evaluation   187
10.1 Introduction   187
10.2 Insertion gain measurement   187
10.3 Functional gain measurement   190
10.4 Speech audiometry   191
10.5 Subjective evaluation   197
10.6 Summary   199
     References   199
     Further reading   200

11 Client management and rehabilitation   201
11.1 The rehabilitation process   201
11.2 Practical aspects of rehabilitation   207
11.3 Assistive devices for the hearing impaired   213
11.4 Management practices   214
11.5 Improving communications   217
11.6 The role of other specialists   219
11.7 Summary   220
     References   220
     Further reading   221

PART THREE   Special Aspects of Hearing Aid Audiology   223

12 Assessment and management of special problems   225
12.1 Tinnitus   225
     References for section 12.1   232
     Further reading for section 12.1   232
12.2 Impedance audiometry   232
     Further reading for section 12.2   240
12.3 Specialized audiometric tests   240
     References for section 12.3   246
     Further reading for section 12.3   246
12.4 Non-organic hearing loss   246

References for section 12.4   249
Further reading for section 12.4   250
12.5 Automatic audiometry   250
References for section 12.5   252
Further reading for section 12.5   252

13 Paediatric provision   **253**
13.1 The effect of hearing loss in children   253
13.2 Habilitation of hearing impaired children   259
13.3 Summary   264
References   264
Further reading   265

Appendix   Glossary   266
Index   277

Foreword

Both for those in training towards qualification in hearing aid audiology and for those simply wishing to revise and update their knowledge, it is a perennial problem to acquire one book which provides comprehensive and up-to-date material on hearing aid audiology. *Principles of Hearing Aid Audiology* meets the need for a text book which deals not only with the foundation sciences of hearing aid audiology but also the many and varied aspects of audiological practice where the objective is the rehabilitation of the hearing impaired through hearing aid prescription and fitting. In bringing together all the material contained in this book, Maryanne Tate has drawn on her considerable experience in the training of hearing aid audiologists as well as in dealing with the hearing impaired themselves. As a result, this book has total relevance to the needs of the many professional groups whose work brings them into contact with the hearing impaired.

The very practical nature of hearing aid audiology is fully recognized so that the purely theoretical aspects are presented and explained with a view to supporting hearing aid audiology in practice. With so many audiology text books emanating from the USA, *Principles of Hearing Aid Audiology* will, I am sure, be greatly welcomed by readers in the UK. Undoubtedly, this book will feature prominently on any list of recommended reading in audiology and, at the same time, will serve as a very useful work of reference.

Barry Downes, LLB, FSHAA
Registrar of the Society of
Hearing Aid Audiologists, 1988–1993

Acknowledgements

Many colleagues and friends have helped and encouraged me to write this book. Dr Mark Lutman (Institute of Hearing Research, Nottingham) provided both critical comments and encouragement when I needed them in the early stages, and I am particularly grateful for the contributions of:

Dr Loraine Lawrence, S.C.M.O. Audiological Medicine, Tameside Area Health Services

Mr Joseph Rumble, Consultant Oral Surgeon, North Middlesex Hospital

Mr Peter Grimaldi, Consultant ENT Surgeon, St Mary's Hospital, Isle of Wight

Mr Robert Rendell, Training Officer, Hidden Hearing Ltd, and Registrar of the Society of Hearing Aid Audiologists

Dr Derek Tate, Associate Head of Centre for Design, Manufacture and Technology, University College Salford.

I appreciate the assistance given by Roy Sands (Special Projects Manager, Rayovac UK Ltd) and Julian Parmenter (Technical Sales Manager, Duracell UK Ltd) with regard to battery specifications. I should also like to express my sincere thanks to all those who read and commented on part, or all, of the manuscript, especially Neville Browne (Director, The London Otological Centre), Keith Attenborough (Professor of Acoustics, The Open University), Barry Downes (Managing Director, SieTech Hearing Ltd), David Gaszczyk (Audiologist, BMI Healthcare), John Millership and Alan Hall (Hearing Aid Audiologists, Amplivox and Ultratone Ltd).

Finally my thanks must go to Dorothy Rothwell who word-processed the manuscript and tolerated my many revisions without complaint, John Beeton and other colleagues and friends who helped me in many ways, and to all those friends and family who endured my preoccupation throughout 1992 and 1993, especially my children Kerry, Joanne, Christopher and Russell.

PART ONE
Fundamental Sciences

Acoustics 1

1.1 PHYSICAL PROPERTIES OF SOUND

1.1.1 SOUND GENERATION

Sound requires a source, a medium through which to travel and a detector. The detector is usually a listener but could be a sound measuring device, a sound level meter.

Sound is generated by a vibrating object and is transmitted through a medium or substance, which is generally air, but may be any elastic medium: gas, liquid or solid. In air, the sound source sets the air particles into vibration, in the same back and forth motion as that of the vibrating sound source. The medium itself is not transferred to the detector, as each particle is displaced only a very small distance from its resting position (equilibrium). The energy is passed across the medium as a series of compressions and rarefactions (Figure 1.1). This constitutes a sound wave. In compressions, the air particles move closer together and the air pressure is slightly higher than normal; in rarefaction, the particles move away from each other and the air pressure is slightly lower than normal.

The speed of sound varies with the density of the medium through which it travels. The denser the medium, the faster sound travels. Sound becomes weaker with increasing distance from the source. If there are no obstacles to affect the progress of the sound waves, the decrease in intensity will be in accordance with the **inverse square law**. This states that the intensity varies inversely with the square of the distance from the sound source (Figure 1.2).

1.1.2 PROPERTIES OF SOUND

The simplest wave form is a sine wave, or sinusoid. A sine wave is produced by simple harmonic motion, where each vibration is repeated

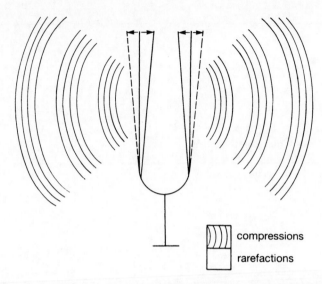

Fig. 1.1 The tines of the tuning fork move alternately towards and apart from each other causing alternate regions of compression and rarefaction that move outwards through the air.

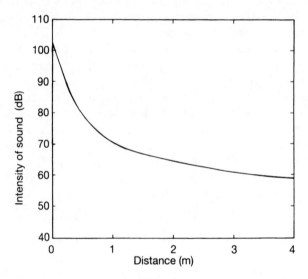

Fig. 1.2 As distance away from the sound source increases, the sound level falls, in accordance with the inverse square law.

back and forth. This motion repeats itself exactly in equal periods of time and is known as periodic motion. Sine waves are very clean or pure sounds and are therefore termed simple or pure tones. A pure tone can be described by three characteristics: frequency, intensity and duration.

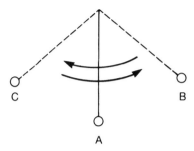

Fig. 1.3 A complete cycle of the pendulum is shown by movement from A to B, from B to C and from C back to A.

(a) Frequency

The frequency of a sound is denoted by the number of cycles of vibration that occur in 1 second. A cycle consists of one compression and one rarefaction of air particles. It can perhaps be better visualized as the movement of a pendulum. In a complete cycle, the pendulum would move from its resting position A to a position to one side B, then back through the resting position A to the other side C, and back to the resting position (Figure 1.3).

If it takes 1 second to complete one full cycle, the frequency is 1 cycle per second (cps), or 1 hertz (Hz); 10 Hz, therefore, means 10 cps. Cycles per second are termed hertz after Heinrich Hertz, a nineteenth-century German physicist. The more cycles that occur in one second, the higher is the frequency of the sound. A stringed instrument can readily be heard to produce a higher frequency as the strings are shortened.

Pitch is the subjective attribute of frequency and is closely related to frequency. The higher frequency, the higher the pitch. However, as pitch is subjective, it cannot be measured directly.

The piano produces its lowest note at 27.5 Hz and its highest at 4186 Hz; Middle C is 261.63 Hz (Somerfield, 1987). The human ear can detect a much wider frequency range than this and the young healthy ear can perceive a frequency range from approximately 20 Hz to 20 000 Hz. Sounds below this frequency range are called infrasonic, and those above this range are called ultrasonic.

Wavelength is inversely proportional to frequency. The wavelength is measured as the distance covered by one complete cycle. As frequency increases, wavelength decreases.

Wavelength can be determined using the formula:

$$\text{Wavelength } (\lambda) = \frac{\text{speed}}{\text{frequency}}$$

The speed of sound in air is approximately 340 metres per second. So, for example, if the frequency of a sound wave is 550 Hz, the wavelength in air will be:

$$\frac{340\,\text{m/s}}{550\,\text{Hz}} = 0.6\,\text{m}$$

(b) Period

The time required for **one** cycle is known as the period (Figure 1.4). The relationship between frequency and period can be expressed as:

$$\text{Frequency (f)} = \frac{1}{\text{Period}}$$

(c) Intensity

Intensity is defined as the amount of energy transmitted per second per unit area.

In the SI system, energy per second is measured in joules per second (J/s) or watts (W), area is measured in square metres (m²), therefore the unit of intensity is the watt per square metre (W/m²).

Frequently, we measure the sound pressure level at a given point and not the intensity, although it can be shown that, in free-field conditions, the intensity is proportional to the square of the pressure:

$$\text{Intensity} \propto (\text{pressure})^2$$

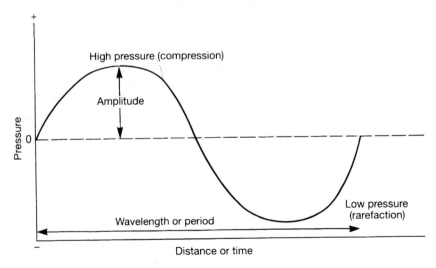

Fig. 1.4 One cycle of a pure tone.

This is a little beyond the scope of this book so, to avoid confusion, we will consider only the sound pressure level. Sound pressure level is the amount of pressure variation about the mean ('amplitude' in Figure 1.4). The greater the force or energy applied to the vibrating body, the more intense the vibrations. The intensity is governed by the distance the air particles move from their place of rest. With increased force, they will move further and thus cause increased compressions and rarefactions. In the SI system, pressure is expressed in pascals (Pa).

A vibrating source sets up tiny changes in air pressure. These changes are so small they are measured in terms of micro pascals (μPa), which are millionths of a pascal. The human ear is sensitive to pressure changes from 20 μPa to 20 Pa. In other words, the greatest pressure change the human ear can withstand is a million times greater than that which is just audible.

Since the range of hearing is so great, the numbers involved are very large and it is more convenient to describe intensity using a logarithmic scale, the decibel scale. Decibels (dB) are units of relative intensity. The number of dB describes how much greater is the intensity of a measured sound than a fixed reference level. The dBSPL scale (decibels sound pressure level), for example, uses 0.00002 Pa as its fixed reference level, so that 0 dBSPL = 0.00002 Pa.

0 dBSPL approximates to the **minimum** audible sound pressure at 1 kHz
30 dBSPL approximates to a whisper
60 dBSPL approximates to quiet conversation
90 dBSPL approximates to shout
120 dBSPL is uncomfortably loud for most people

Decibels are considered in more detail in section 1.2.

1.1.3 COMPLEX SOUNDS

Pure tones can be produced artificially using a tuning fork or an electronic sine-wave generator, but they rarely occur naturally. Most sounds consist of a number of different tones, although these can be broken down into the component pure tones using frequency analysis. Each component pure tone may vary in amplitude, frequency and phase.

1.1.4 PHASE

When we consider the phase of a sinusoidal wave, we are stating the position at any point in the cycle.

Any circle corresponds to 360° rotation. The degrees of rotation are used to denote the course of travel, where 0° is the starting point, 90° is

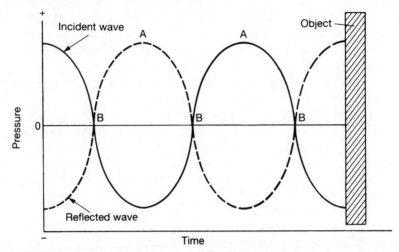

Fig. 1.5 Two pure tones of equal frequency and intensity, which are out of phase by 180°. This creates standing waves in which occur areas with increased sound (A) and areas without sound (B).

a quarter of the way around the circle, 180° is half-way and so on. Tones are exactly out of phase if they differ from the standard starting point by 180°. Figure 1.5 illustrates tones that are out of phase.

1.1.5 PERIODIC SOUNDS

Complex sounds may have a waveform that repeats itself over time. Such sounds are called periodic. Periodic sounds are musical or harmonic.

The lowest frequency of the tones presented determines the fundamental frequency. The pitch of a note is recognized by its fundamental frequency. Thus Middle C, for example, can be recognized regardless of whether it is played on a piano or a violin.

In a periodic sound, all frequencies present are harmonics. These are whole number multiples (integers) of the fundamental frequency. A 1 kHz tone has harmonics at 2 kHz, 3 kHz, 4 kHz and so on, although not all the harmonics are necessarily present. Two instruments playing the same note sound different because their sound contains different harmonics, although the fundamental frequency remains the same. Harmonics are referred to by number. The fundamental frequency is the first harmonic (1 × 1). The second harmonic is twice the fundamental, the third harmonic is three times the fundamental. The fundamental frequency does not necessarily have to be heard for recognition. Our minds can determine the fundamental from the pattern of harmonics.

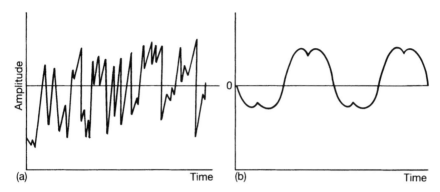

Fig. 1.6 Waveforms of noise and periodic sound: (a) an aperiodic (or noise) waveform; (b) a periodic waveform.

1.1.6 APERIODIC SOUNDS

Aperiodic or non-periodic sounds do not have a regularly repeating waveform. They consist of more than one frequency and are not harmonically related. This random and unstable waveform has no stated period or repetition and is perceived as noise (Figure 1.6). Certain particular types of noise may be used in audiometry:

- White noise consists of all the frequencies of the audible spectrum present at equal intensities.
- Pink noise consists of equal energy per octave. This produces a lower frequency noise than white noise since each octave contains equal energy but a varying number of frequencies. For example, the octave 250 Hz to 500 Hz contains 250 discrete frequencies, whereas the octave 2 kHz to 4 kHz contains 2000 discrete frequencies; yet each of these contains the same amount of energy.

1.1.7 WAVE MOTION

In an environment where there is no interference from reflections (a 'free-field'), sound waves will spread longitudinally and gradually lose energy as they move away from the sound source.

The intensity of the sound decreases proportionally to the square of the distance from the sound source. This is the **inverse square law** (Figure 1.2) and in practice it means that a doubling of distance will produce a reduction of 6 dB in the sound pressure level.

In an enclosed field, hard surfaces will reflect sound waves. Sound reflections can increase the sound level within a room, making it easier to hear, as long as the reflections follow the original sound very rapidly. When the time between the incident wave (sound source) and the

reflection is prolonged to a degree that is noticeable, it is termed reverberation. A reflected sound that occurs some time after the original is
heard as an echo. When a reflection follows closely, it adds to the
direct sound; reverberation follows with a short time delay, which may
be destructive to intelligibility; with a greater be delay, a distinct echo
may be heard. This may be illustrated as follows:

> Reflection   reverberation   echo
>   Reflection   reverberation   echo

In a large, empty room, the reverberation effect may last for several
seconds, which will make speech indistinct. Soft furnishings will absorb
and help to reduce reverberation. Reverberation is particularly destructive to intelligibility for hearing aid users. It is not, however, desirable
to cut out all reflection (except for research purposes, as in an anechoic
chamber) as this makes the room very quiet and 'dead'.

Standing waves are caused when incident waves and reflected waves
meet and combine to affect the sound level at that particular point. The
interference that this creates may be constructive (increase the sound
level) or destructive (decrease the sound level) (Figure 1.5). When a
standing wave is formed within the confines of an object, resonance
occurs as, for example, in a pipe or in the ear canal. The length of the
pipe or canal will affect the frequency of the standing waves formed
within it. For example, if the length of a pipe is halved, the fundamental frequency of the air column within it is doubled and the
resonant frequency will rise by one octave.

1.1.8 WARBLE TONES

Warble tones are often used in free-field audiometry to reduce the risk
of standing waves affecting test results.

A warble tone is a frequency modulated tone. The tone has a base or
centre frequency, around which it varies. For example, a 1 kHz warble
tone might vary from 950 Hz to 1050 Hz, which would be a frequency
deviation of ±50 Hz, or 5%. The tone therefore consists of frequencies
above and below its centre frequency, and it changes rapidly between
these limits. The number of frequency changes in one second is termed
the 'modulation rate'.

1.2 THE MEASUREMENT OF SOUND

1.2.1 DECIBEL SCALES

The decibel scales express a ratio between two numbers.

Most quantities are measured in terms of fixed units, so, for example, when we say that the distance between two points is 10 m, we mean the distance is ten times greater than 1 m. Logarithms are used as a convenient method of expressing the ratio. A logarithm (log) tells how many times the base number is multiplied by itself, 10^2 means 10 to the power of 2, that is, 10 is multiplied by itself once, and 10^3 is multiplied by itself twice, as follows:

$10^1 = 10$ therefore $\log_{10}(10) = 1$
$10^2 = 10 \times 10$ therefore $\log_{10}(100) = 2$
$10^3 = 10 \times 10 \times 10$ therefore $\log_{10}(1000) = 3$

The wide range of intensities involved is compressed by transforming it to a logarithmic scale. The unit of relative intensity is the bel, named after Alexander Graham Bell, who first patented the telephone. One bel equals ten decibels. The bel is rather too large a unit to reflect the accuracy required for audiometry. In measuring sound intensity or sound pressure level, the decibel scale is therefore used.

Any tenfold increase in sound pressure corresponds to 20 dB. For example, a noise level of 80 dB has a sound pressure that is 1000 times greater (10^3) than a noise of 20 dB. Subjectively, 10 dB appears as a doubling of loudness, whereas 1 dB is equivalent to the smallest change of intensity we can detect in ideal conditions.

In mathematical terms, we can see that:

$$\text{dBSPL} = 20 \log_{10} \frac{P_1}{P_{\text{ref}}}$$

where P_1 = measured pressure
and P_{ref} = the audiological reference pressure.

The audiological reference pressure is 0.00002 pascals. So, for example, if:

$$P_1 = 0.002 \, \text{Pa}$$

and

$$P_{\text{ref}} = 0.00002 \, \text{Pa}$$

using the formula

$$\text{dBSPL} = 20 \log_{10} \frac{P_1}{P_{\text{ref}}}$$

gives us

$$20 \log_{10} \frac{0.002}{0.00002}$$

$$= 20 \log_{10} \frac{100}{1}$$

$$= 20 \times 2 = 40 \, \text{dB}$$

since the log of 100 to base 10 = 2

For those who are less able mathematically, it may be helpful to show the relationship between dBSPL and pascals as follows:

Sound pressure level: dBSPL	Sound pressure: Pa	Equivalent to:
120	= 20.0	Discomfort
100	= 2.0	Pneumatic drill
80	= 0.2	Shouting
60	= 0.02	Quiet conversation
40	= 0.002	Loud whispering
20	= 0.0002	Rustling leaves
0	= 0.00002	(Standard audiological reference)

The range of pressures to which the average normally hearing person is sensitive starts at 0 dBSPL (0.00002 Pa) and has a limit, where sound becomes uncomfortably loud, of 120 dBSPL (20 Pa). This range is called the dynamic range of hearing.

Since decibels express a ratio between two sound pressures, their values in dB cannot simply be added together. Two sound sources of 40 dBSPL, for example, do not equal 80 dBSPL; in fact, this results in an increase of 3 dB, producing 43 dBSPL overall.

To be meaningful, a ratio must have a reference level. It is pointless to say that a sound is ten times greater, unless we also state what it is greater than. In audiometry, a number of different dB scales are used and each has its own reference level. For example, the **dBSPL** scale (dB sound pressure level) expresses the pressure of a sound in relation to the standard audiological reference pressure, 0.00002 Pa, which is the minimum pressure required to cause the sensation of hearing in the midfrequency region. The dBSPL scale compares with a flat or 'absolute' reference: it takes no account of the way hearing varies with frequency.

Other decibel scales used include dB(A), dB(B), dB(C), dB(D) and dBHL. A range of scales are used because the human ear is not equally sensitive at all frequencies or intensities. The different decibel scales attempt to reflect these changes. For audiometric purposes dB(A) and dBHL scales are important. The dBHL scale is used when sounds are presented monaurally through air conduction headphones or bone conduction transducers. The dB(A) scale is used when the sound level is presented 'free-field' in a room. The two scales are very similar, but the dB(A) scale provides values that are about 4 dB greater than dBHL values.

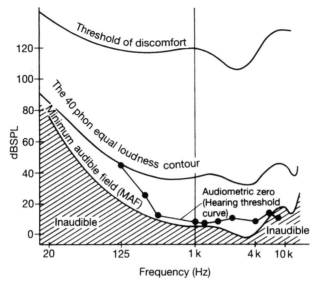

Fig. 1.7 A diagrammatic representation of the dynamic range of human hearing.

The SPL (sound pressure level) values for audiometric zero (0 dBHL) at each frequency are given in BS 2497: Part 5 (1988). The values are the recommended equivalent threshold sound pressure levels (RETSPL) in a 9 A acoustic coupler. The RETSPL values provide average minimum audible pressure (MAP) under headphones, which may be illustrated as a hearing threshold curve (Figure 1.7), or a table providing values at the various audiometric frequencies (Table 1.1).

Table 1.1 Recommended reference equivalent threshold sound pressure levels (RETSPL) in a 9 A coupler (British Standards Institution, 1988)

Frequency Hz	RETSPL dB (Reference: 20 μPa)
125	45.0
250	25.5
500	11.5
1 k	7.0
2 k	9.0
3 k	10.0
4 k	9.5
6 k	15.5
8 k	13.0
Pattern of earphone	Telephonics TDH39 with MX41/ AR cushion

The values were established on the basis of a statistical average obtained by testing many otologically normal people between the ages of 18 and 30 years. A similar method was used to obtain the Minimum Audible Field (MAF) which sets out thresholds obtained binaurally, in response to sound pressures presented through loudspeakers. Thresholds taken from the MAF curve are an average of about 6 dB more sensitive than the normal MAP thresholds.

1.2.2 THE SOUND LEVEL METER

A sound level meter is a precision instrument used for sound measurement. A precision microphone converts the sound signal to an electrical signal, which is amplified by a pre-amplifier before being processed. The signal may be displayed in linear dBSPL, or it may pass through a weighting network. This is an electronic circuit that varies in sensitivity across the frequency range, to simulate the sensitivity of the human ear (Figure 1.8).

The weighting networks are termed A, B, C and D. The A weighting network corresponds to an inverted equal loudness contour (section 1.4.2) at low sound pressure levels. The B network corresponds to medium SPLs and the C network to high SPLs. The D network is used for aircraft noise measurements.

1.3 THE AUDIOMETER

1.3.1 THE AUDIOMETER AND ITS CALIBRATION

Hearing is a subjective sensation and therefore cannot truly be 'measured'. Audiometry measures the **stimulus** which causes the sensation of hearing.

An audiometer is an instrument of comparison, which indicates the difference between the sound pressure level required to produce hear-

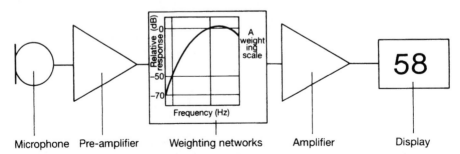

Fig. 1.8 Constituent parts of a sound level meter using the A weighting network.

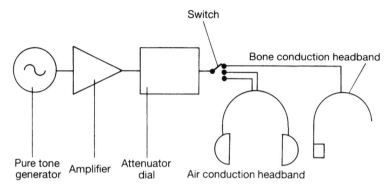

Fig. 1.9 Constituent parts of an audiometer.

ing in the individual under test and that required to produce hearing in an average normal young person. An audiometer generates pure tones at specified points within a restricted range of frequencies considered important for communication, usually the octave intervals from 125 Hz to 8 kHz.

An octave is a doubling of frequency. Most audiometers also produce tones at the half-octave intervals, 750 Hz, 1.5 kHz, 3 kHz and 6 kHz. The sound level can also be varied, usually in 5 dB steps, from −10 dBHL to 110 dBHL or more. The duration of the tones is controlled by an interruptor switch. The audiometer is provided with two transducers, a pair of headphones and a bone vibrator. A block diagram of a basic audiometer is shown in Figure 1.9.

An audiometer must be accurate to be of value and, to this end, all audiometers are calibrated to British Standards when new and the calibration should be re-checked at least once a year. BS 5966 (1980) defines the aspects of pure-tone audiometer accuracy with which manufacturers should comply.

The main points of this standard, for our purposes, can be summarized as follows:

- Frequency accuracy must be ±3%.
- Purity must be such that the total harmonic distortion does not exceed 5% (for air conduction).
- The attenuator 5 dB steps must be correct within ±1 dB.
- Unwanted sound from the audiometer should be inaudible up to and including the dial setting 50 dBHL.
- The narrow band noise filters must be centred on the frequency (according to a given table).
- The rise and fall times of the signal tone should be within specification (section 1.3.3).

- The hearing level must be accurate to within ±3 dB from 125 Hz to 4 kHz and to within ±5 dB at 6 kHz and 8 kHz.

Laboratory calibration is carried out for the complete audiometer. The transducers (headphones and bone vibrator) are a part of the audiometer and should not be exchanged unless the audiometer is recalibrated with the new transducers.

In addition to calibration, the audiometer should be checked daily as follows:

1.3.2 DAILY AUDIOMETER CHECKS

- Straighten any tangled leads. Ensure that all connections are firm and giving good contact. Flex the leads for possible intermittency.
- Check that all knobs and switches are secure and function in a silent, smooth and click-free manner.
- Check function of response button.
- Check tension of AC and BC headbands.
- Check output levels for all tones at 10–15 dB above own known threshold for AC (each earphone) and BC. Your own audiogram should be used for this approximate calibration check.
- Check at 60 dBHL for all tones on AC (each earphone) for noticeable distortion, intermittency, etc. Repeat at 40 dBHL for BC.
- Check masking noise over a range of outputs, also loudness balance and other facilities, if to be used.
- Check battery condition, if appropriate.
- Generally ensure that the audiometer and all its attachments are clean. Wipe earphones and BC receiver with clean, dry tissues.

1.3.3 RISE AND FALL TIMES

The audiometer output signal is not an instantaneous event. The signal rises until it reaches its maximum and falls off in a similar manner when the tone is switched off (Figure 1.10).

Rise time is defined as the time taken for the signal to rise from −60 dB (or −20 dB) to within 1 dB of its steady state. The time taken for the signal to rise from −60 dB to −1 dB of its steady state should not be more than 200 milliseconds. The time taken for the signal to rise from −20 dB to −1 dB of its steady state should be at least 20 milliseconds. (BS 5966: 1980).

Fall time is defined as the time taken for the signal to decay by 60 dB from its steady state. Fall time should not exceed 200 milliseconds, nor be less than 20 milliseconds. (BS 5966: 1980).

This rise and fall (decay) should be correctly timed or it may affect the results of the audiometric test:

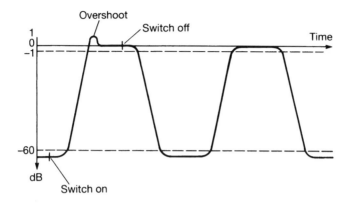

Fig. 1.10 The rise and fall envelope of test tones. Between the dotted lines sound should rise or fall in a progressive manner. (After BS 5966 (1980).)

- Too slow a rise time may result in erroneously poor thresholds, because this does not elicit the maximum on-effect of the ear.
- Too brief a rise time produces an overshoot which may be heard as a click. This may result in erroneously good thresholds if the patient responds to the click rather than the test tone. An overshoot should never be greater than 1 dB.

1.4 THE PSYCHOLOGICAL PROPERTIES OF SOUND

1.4.1 PSYCHOACOUSTICS

The study of the psychological properties of sound is known as psychoacoustics.

The way in which we hear sound is subjective and cannot be directly measured. Subjective qualities are compared with reference levels obtained by averaging the judgements of a large number of normally-hearing people.

1.4.2 LOUDNESS

Loudness is the subjective perception of sound in terms of intensity. The relative loudness of pure tones is normally expressed as equal loudness contours. Each contour represents sounds that appear equally loud. Each contour or curve has a loudness value given in phons, which can be defined as the sound pressure level of a 1 kHz tone judged to be of equal loudness.

The 40 phon curve, for example (Figure 1.7), represents pure tones across the frequency range, which are judged equally loud as a 1 kHz tone at an intensity of 40 dBSPL. An inverted 40 phon curve is used for the A weighting scale of a sound level meter.

Another unit of loudness, the sone, is used for the purpose of providing a scale to define loudness. This numerical scale of loudness is based on judgements of average listeners as to when sounds are 'twice as loud' or 'half as loud'. One sone is taken to be the loudness of a 1 kHz tone at 40 dBSPL. Thus, 1 sone has a loudness level of 40 phons. A sound which has a loudness of 2 sones is one which is judged to be twice as loud.

In terms of sound pressure level, an increase of 10 dB corresponds to a doubling of loudness.

1.4.3 PITCH

Pitch is the subjective perception of sound in terms of frequency. The unit of pitch used is the mel. One thousand mels represents the pitch of a 1 kHz tone presented at 40 phons. The ability to recognize the pitch of sounds of different frequencies is known as 'frequency resolution'. The average normal person can discriminate a frequency difference where a change of 3 Hz occurs, although this varies across the audible spectrum.

1.4.4 TEMPORAL INTEGRATION

The effect of duration on the recognition of sound is known as 'temporal integration'. Tone presentations that are very brief may not be heard. The shorter a tone presentation, the more intense must be that sound if it is to be perceived. Duration also has an effect on the apparent pitch of a sound. Tones that are of very short duration will be perceived as a click.

Sensorineural hearing loss may reduce the ability to discriminate pitch. It may also increase the sensation of loudness, such that a small increase in objective intensity results in a large increase in subjective loudness. This abnormal loudness growth is termed recruitment.

1.5 SUMMARY

For sound to exist it must be in our audible frequency range, which is normally 20–20 000 Hz, and there must be an elastic medium to convey the vibrations.

Simple harmonic motion produces a pure tone, which is a sound of one frequency. Sound is created by a vibrating object, which produces alternate compressions and rarefactions in the medium, which is usually air.

The frequency of vibration is calculated by the number of vibrations, or cycles, in 1 second. The time taken for 1 cycle is known as the period. The unit of frequency is hertz; 1 Hz = 1 cycle per second.

All sound can be broken down into its component pure tones. The decibel scale is used to describe the amplitude of sound. Decibels are not absolute units of measurement but provide a ratio between a measured quantity and an agreed reference level, which must be specified.

An audiometer provides a comparison between the hearing of the subject under test and average normal hearing as set out in the relevant British Standard. Audiometers must be regularly checked and calibrated to ensure accuracy.

Sound can be measured objectively in terms of frequency, intensity or pressure, and duration. Hearing is subjective and may be described in terms of pitch and loudness.

REFERENCES

British Standards Institution (1980) *BS 5966: Specification for Audiometers*, British Standards Institution, London.

British Standards Institution (1988) *BS 2497: Part 5: Standard Reference Zero for the Calibration of Pure-Tone Air Conduction Audiometers*, British Standards Institution, London.

Somerfield, Q. (1987) *The Musician's Guide to Acoustics*, Dent, London.

FURTHER READING

Foreman, J.E.K. (1990) *Sound Analysis and Noise Control*, Van Nostrand Reinhold, New York.

Moore, B.C.J. (1989) *An Introduction to the Psychology of Hearing*, 3rd edn, Academic Press, London.

Pickles, J.D. (1988) *An Introduction to the Physiology of Hearing*, 2nd edn, Academic Press, London.

Speaks, C.E. (1992) *Introduction to Sound*, Chapman & Hall, London.

Anatomy and physiology of the ear

2

2.1 ANATOMY OF THE EAR

The ear (Figure 2.1) can be thought of as consisting of three parts, known as the outer, the middle and the inner ear.

2.1.1 THE OUTER EAR

The outer or external ear is divided into two parts: the pinna or auricle, and the external auditory meatus.

(a) The pinna

The first part of the external ear is the pinna or auricle. This is formed of irregular-shaped cartilage covered by firmly adherent skin. The dependent lobule is mainly fat. Anteriorly the cartilage forms the tragus, which covers the entrance of the external auditory meatus. The main anatomical features of the pinna are shown in Figure 2.2. Attached to the pinna are three vestigial muscles, all supplied by the facial nerve. In some animals they function to direct the pinna towards the direction of a sound source, in humans they are mostly redundant.

(b) The external auditory meatus

The cartilage of the pinna extends inwards to form the first one-third of the external auditory meatus (ear canal). This horizontal curved canal (Figure 2.3) is usually about 2.5 cm long in an adult. It is closed at its medial end by the tympanic membrane (eardrum). The outer one-third curves inwards, slightly upwards and backwards, and is lined by skin richly endowed with hairs and apocrine (sweat), sebaceous (oil) and

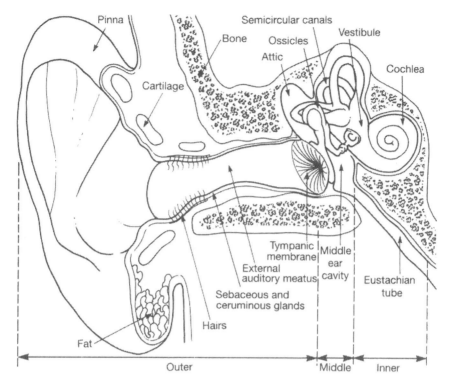

Fig. 2.1 The outer, middle and inner ear.

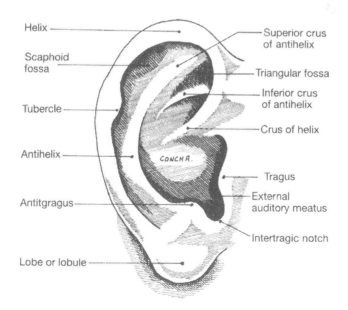

Fig. 2.2 Anatomical features of a left pinna.

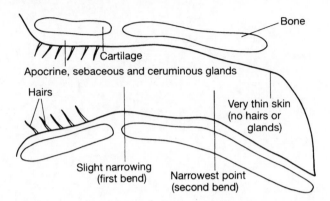

Fig. 2.3 Diagrammatic representation of the external auditory meatus.

ceruminous (wax) glands. The inner two-thirds of the canal is bony, formed from the squamous temporal bone. This part of the canal runs downwards and forwards and is lined with thin, closely adherent skin, largely devoid of hairs and glands. About 5 mm from the tympanic membrane the floor of the canal dips to form a recess; debris often collects here and is difficult to remove.

The external ear has an extensive sensory nerve supply from branches of three cranial nerves (V, VII and X). The inner part of the canal is particularly sensitive and can produce a cough reflex when stimulated due to its innervation from the tenth cranial nerve (Vagus).

It is important to remember the close proximity to the external auditory meatus of three cranial structures: the mastoid air cells (behind), the middle cranial fossa (above) and the temporomandibular (jaw) joint (in front). Injury or infection in the canal can extend to involve these.

2.1.2. THE MIDDLE EAR CLEFT

The middle ear cleft is made up of five anatomical parts: the tympanic cavity, the auditory or Eustachian tube, the aditus, the mastoid antrum and the mastoid air cells.

(a) The tympanic cavity

The tympanic cavity is the part of the middle ear cleft which is usually thought of as 'the middle ear'. It is separated from the external ear by the tympanic membrane (eardrum), and from the internal ear by the round and oval windows. It has connections with the nasopharynx via the Eustachian tube and with the mastoid cavity via the aditus. It

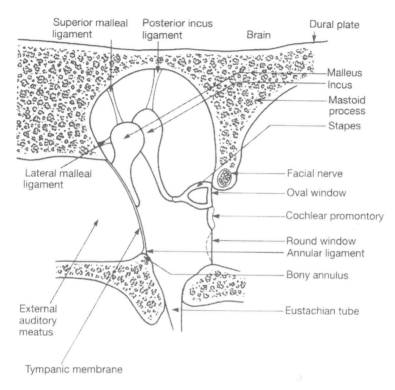

Fig. 2.4 Diagrammatic representation of the tympanic cavity.

houses the ossicles and their muscular attachments and has many important anatomical landmarks.

The cavity (Figure 2.4) may be thought of as a narrow room, the height and length of which is about 15 mm, with medial and lateral walls which curve inwards towards the centre; this makes them about 2 mm apart in the middle and 6 mm apart at the roof.

The lateral wall is formed mainly by the tympanic membrane. This translucent membrane is set obliquely, such that the roof and posterior wall of the external auditory meatus are shorter than the floor and anterior wall. The membrane consists of three layers, that is, a middle, incomplete, fibrous layer, which is covered with skin on the outer surface, and the mucous membrane of the middle ear cavity on the inner surface. The area of drum containing the fibrous layer is known as the pars tensa (Figure 2.5), and where this is deficient, the pars flaccida. The handle of the first auditory ossicle, the malleus, is attached in the centre of the pars tensa on the medial surface and produces a small elevation on the drum, easily seen with an otoscope.

The medial wall separates the middle from the inner ear. It has a

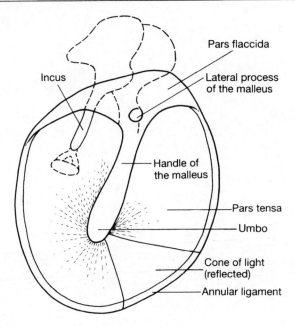

Fig. 2.5 Right tympanic membrane. Broken lines indicate the ossicles in the middle ear cavity.

central bulge, the promontory, which is formed by the first turn of the cochlea. Above and behind the promontory lies the oval window which is closed by the footplate of the stapes, the third of the auditory ossicles. This window separates the middle ear from the scala vestibuli of the cochlea. Below and behind the promontory is the round window which separates the middle ear from the scala tympani; this is closed by a fibrous disc. The seventh cranial nerve (facial) passes across the medial wall, lying in a bony canal above the promontory.

The anterior wall has two important landmarks:

- The opening of the Eustachian tube which connects the middle ear with the nasopharynx.
- The bony canal for the tensor tympani muscle. This muscle attaches to the malleus and tenses the eardrum. The tensor tympani is innervated by the fifth (trigeminal) cranial nerve.

High up on the posterior wall is the aditus, which connects the middle ear cavity with the mastoid antrum. Below this is the pyramid, a projection of bone from which the second muscle of the middle ear, the stapedius, arises. This muscle is attached to the third ossicle, the stapes, and is supplied with motor fibres from the seventh nerve (facial), which passes down this wall. A branch of the seventh nerve, the chorda tympani, comes out through a small hole lateral to the

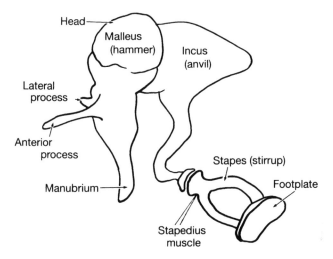

Fig. 2.6 The middle ear ossicles.

pyramid. A further description of the middle ear muscles will be found in section 12.2.7.

The roof separates the cavity from the middle cranial fossa and is formed from a thin plate of the petrous temporal bone. The floor is again only a thin plate of bone. Below and behind is the jugular foramen, through which passes the major vein of the head and neck. Below and in front is the canal containing the carotid artery.

This four-walled 'room' is normally filled with air and contains the three auditory ossicles (Figure 2.6) that serve to transmit sound energy from the tympanic membrane across the middle ear cavity to the cochlea. The first, the malleus (hammer), is attached to the tympanic membrane laterally and articulates with the incus (anvil) medially. The incus has a body and two processes, one of which articulates with the stapes, the other rests on the posterior wall. Finally the part of the stapes (stirrup), known as the footplate, closes the oval window and therefore communicates with the perilymph of the cochlea. The two middle ear muscles, the tensor tympani and the stapedius, have already been described; these modify the transmission of sound energy across the ossicular chain.

As with the external auditory meatus, it is very important to remember the close proximity of the middle ear cleft to several important anatomical structures: the temporal lobe of the brain lies above, and behind is the cerebellum, both separated only by a layer of bone; the facial nerve passes through the cleft in a bony canal, which may be very thin; both major vessels of the head and neck, the carotid artery and the jugular vein, run close to the floor of the cleft; and, of course, lying medially, is the inner ear. All these are susceptible to spread of infection or disease from the middle ear.

(b) The Eustachian tube

In an adult, the Eustachian tube is about 3.5 cm long. It connects the nasopharynx with the tympanic cavity and in health provides regular ventilation of the middle ear. It also, however, provides a pathway for disease to spread from the nose and throat to the ear. It is normally closed at rest but opens temporarily during yawning or swallowing. At its lower end it is formed of cartilage and membrane and opens behind the nasal cavity; it then passes upwards and outwards and enters the tympanic cavity. This upper one-third of the tube is bony. In a young child the Eustachian tube is shorter, wider and more horizontal, and is much more prone to dysfunction.

(c) The mastoid antrum and mastoid air cells

A short tube, the aditus, leads from the back of the tympanic cavity to the mastoid antrum.

The antrum is a cavity within the part of the bony skull known as the petrous temporal bone. It communicates posteriorly through several openings with the mastoid air cells (Figure 2.7). The number and size of these cells varies considerably among individuals. The mastoid air cells are very susceptible to spread of disease from the rest of the middle ear cleft.

The whole of the middle ear cleft is lined with a continuous layer of cells (epithelium), some of which provide lubrication (in the Eustachian tube), and others of which are normally flattened and do not produce

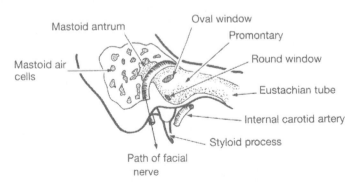

Fig. 2.7 A deep section of the middle ear, showing the mastoid antrum, and the path of the facial nerve.

mucus (for example, in the tympanic cavity). These cells are prone to change in shape and function if the cleft is unhealthy.

2.1.3 THE INNER EAR

The inner ear, known as the labyrinth because of its complicated structure, lies entirely within the temporal bone of the skull. It is comprised of a membranous sac filled with a clear fluid (endolymph) contained within a bony cavity. The space between the sac and the bone is also filled with fluid (perilymph). Endolymph is very similar to intracellular fluid and is therefore high in potassium and low in sodium; conversely, perilymph is similar to cerebrospinal fluid and, as with all extracellular fluid, is high in sodium and low in potassium.

(a) The bony labyrinth

The bony labyrinth is a continuous cavity that communicates function- ally with the middle ear via the oval and round windows. It begins medially with the cochlea, which is about 1 mm wide at its base and 5 mm high, and is best understood by considering the shell of a snail. Looking into the empty shell it is a tube which twists around a central pillar; the cochlea does exactly this, spiralling around a central bony pillar, the modiolus, for two and three-quarter turns. From the modiolus a narrow plate of bone, the spiral lamina, projects into the cavity of the tube along its whole length, partly dividing it into an upper and lower chamber. The basal end of the cochlea opens into the middle part of the cavity called the vestibule. There are several openings from the vestibule: two into the middle ear cleft, one closed by the foot of the stapes and its annular ligament (the oval window), the other by a fibrous disc (the round window); five into the three semicircular canals; and one into the intracranial cavity by a bony aqueduct allowing drainage of perilymph into the cerebrospinal fluid.

The semicircular canals lie posteriorly, and each forms two-thirds of a circle. They lie in three planes at right angles to each other; the anterior and posterior canals are set vertically, and the lateral horizontally.

(b) The membranous labyrinth

This saccular membrane (Figure 2.8) forms a series of communicating sacs and ducts lying within the bony labyrinth. The utricle and saccule lie within the vestibule. They communicate with the three semicircular ducts, the Y-shaped endolymphatic duct and the duct of the cochlea. The whole labyrinth is filled with endolymph.

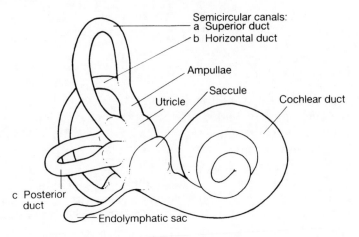

Fig. 2.8 The right membranous labyrinth.

The duct of the cochlea extends along the bony tube lying on the spiral lamina and stretches across to be attached to the outer wall by the spiral ligaments. This forms a triangular-shaped channel with its apex at the modiolus, which effectively forms three chambers within the cochlea (Figure 2.9). The middle chamber formed by the duct, and therefore filled with endolymph, is called the scala media. The upper chamber is called the scala vestibuli and the lower is the scala tympani; as these lie outside the membranous labyrinth they contain perilymph. These two connect at the apex of the cochlea via a small gap, the helicotrema, and at the basal end of the cochlea they end in the vestibule, the scala tympani at the round window and the scala vestibuli at the oval window. The upper wall of the membranous duct is called the vestibular, or Reissner's, membrane, and the lower wall, which extends from the free edge of the spiral lamina, is the basilar membrane. Lining the outer side of the duct is the stria vascularis which maintains the ionic concentration of the endolymph; as the name suggests, this area is very vascular being rich in capillaries.

(c) The organ of Corti

The organ of Corti is a specialized structure of cells that forms the sensory organ of hearing. It is situated within the scala media on the basilar membrane (Figure 2.9).

There are two rows of cells, known as hair cells, which have fine hair-like structures, stereocilia, projecting from their upper surface. These are arranged into an inner row of single hair cells and an outer row of three or four hair cells, separated from each other by a rigid

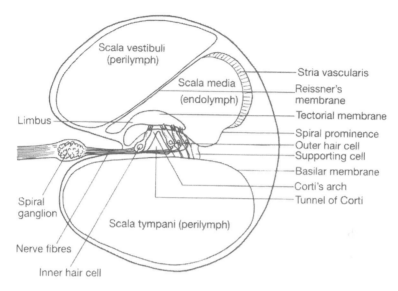

Fig. 2.9 Cross-section of the cochlear duct.

triangular arch called Corti's arch. Within this arch is the cortilymph, a fluid that chemically resembles perilymph. The specialized hair cells are themselves surrounded by various supporting cells. Electron studies have shown the shape of the inner and outer hair cells to be different and also the arrangement of their stereocilia. The inner cells are fatter at the base, resembling a tenpin, and have 70 to 100 stereocilia in two rows forming a double 'V', with the apex directed away from the modiolus. The outer cells are more cylindrical, resembling a test tube, and have more stereocilia, arranged in three rows to form a wide triple 'W'; again the apices are directed away from the modiolus. The stereocilia are not all the same length, the longest being at the apices and gradually reducing in length. Lying over the top of the whole structure is the reticular lamina and above this a gelatinous 'membrane', the tectorial membrane, into which the longest of the stereocilia are embedded having passed through the lamina. The tectorial membrane is attached to the inner side of the cochlea just above the spiral lamina. The estimated number of hair cells is about 3000 to 4000 inner hair cells and about 10 000 to 12 000 outer hair cells.

The shape of the organ of Corti, and the basilar membrane on which it lies, changes along the length of the cochlea, being widest at the apex and becoming progressively narrower towards the base.

The nerve supply to the cochlea is via the eighth cranial nerve (vestibulocochlear). There are both afferent nerves, carrying information to the brain, and efferent nerves, taking information from the brain, serving the cochlea. This is unusual for a sensory organ with no motor function, as efferent nerves are mainly motor; the precise function of these efferent fibres is still being researched (section 2.2.2(a)). They are fewer in number than the afferent fibres; approximately half connect with the inner cells, and half with the outer cells. They differ in that the terminal branches (dendrites) serving the inner hair cells end on the dendrites of the afferent fibres, and those serving the outer cells tend to envelop the base of the cell and its afferent fibres. Each inner hair cell has about 20 afferent nerve fibres synapsing with it, which account for 90–95% of the 30 000 to 40 000 afferent fibres leaving the cochlea. The remaining 5–10% synapse with the outer cells, each fibre being heavily branched and serving up to ten hair cells. The cell bodies of the afferent nerves are found grouped together in the spiral ganglion.

(d) The vestibular organ of balance

Each of the semicircular canals expands into an ampulla at one end. It is here that a special sensory epithelium called the crista is found. A patch of similar epithelium is found at the macula of the utricle and saccule, the former being on a horizontal plane and the latter vertical.

Together these form the vestibular receptor organs. There are two types of specialized cells, type 1 and type 2. Type 1 cells are flask-like and surrounded at the base by a nerve ending shaped like a chalice. Type 2 cells are straighter and more cylindrical with no nerve chalice. Protruding from the cuticular plate is a bundle of sensory 'hairs'. This bundle is comprised of one kinocilium, an additional longer and thicker hair and 50 to 110 stereocilia. These project into a mucus-like substance which is dome-shaped in the ampullae and cylindrical in the utricle; a number of calcareous particles called the otoliths are also contained here. The stereocilia become progressively smaller with increased distance from the kinocilium. This provides both a morphological and functional polarization of the sensory cells. When there is displacement towards the kinocilium the cell is depolarized and produces an increased discharge rate in the afferent nerve fibres; when displaced away from the kinocilium there is a decreased discharge rate.

As with the cochlea there are both afferent and efferent fibres supplying the vestibular sensory cells. These fibres gather together to become the vestibular branch of the eighth nerve.

2.1.4 THE NASOPHARYNX

The pharynx (Figure 2.10) is a fibromuscular tube that forms the upper part of the respiratory and digestive tract; in an adult the whole cavity

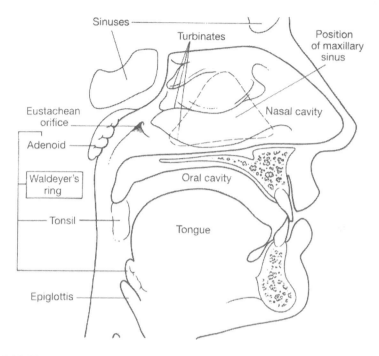

Sinuses
Turbinates
Position of maxillary sinus
Eustachean orifice
Nasal cavity
Adenoid
Waldeyer's ring
Oral cavity
Tonsil
Tongue
Epiglottis

Fig. 2.10 The nasopharynx.

is about 10 cm long. It opens into the nose, mouth and larynx and is thus divided downwards into three parts: the nasopharynx, the oropharynx and the laryngopharynx.

The nasopharynx opens anteriorly into the nasal fossae, bounded above by the base of the skull and below by the soft palate. The lower opening of the Eustachian tube is situated in the lateral wall, and immediately adjacent is the nasopharyngeal tonsil (adenoids). The isthmus of the nasopharynx leads from the oropharynx and is closed during swallowing by raising the soft palate and contracting the palatopharyngeal muscles.

The oropharynx opens anteriorly into the mouth and is bounded above by the soft palate and below by the upper border of the epiglottis. The only major anatomical structures are the palatine tonsils which lie between the muscular faucial pillars on the lateral walls.

The laryngopharynx opens anteriorly into the larynx through a sloping laryngeal inlet. It is bounded above by the epiglottis and below by the cricoid cartilage. The pyriform fossae are small recesses lying on each side bounded by cartilaginous and membranous folds.

Collectively the scattered lymphoid tissue throughout the nasopharynx forms a protective 'ring', known as Waldeyer's ring, which helps prevent the spread of infection into the middle ear and lower respiratory tract.

2.2 THE PHYSIOLOGY OF HEARING

The ear is a remarkable device that is able to detect, collect and encode acoustic information in order to transmit it to the centres of the brain where it can be decoded and utilized by the listerner.

For physiological purposes the ear can be thought of as two functional pieces of apparatus; one that conducts the sound, and another that perceives or 'analyses' the sound reaching it.

2.2.1 THE CONDUCTION OF SOUND

This apparatus consists of the pinna, the external auditory canal, the tympanic membrane, the chain of ossicles and the cochlear fluids.

(a) The pinna

The prime function of the pinna is to act as a sound collection device. It also aids localization of sound in both the horizontal and vertical planes.

The shape of the pinna enables it to funnel the sound towards the external meatus and its forward-tilted angle helps to focus on sound from the front. The pinna also amplifies the sound signal slightly, to a maximum gain of about 10 dB, depending on the frequency of the sound.

Vertical localization is helped by the difference in delay between the main signal and the pinna echoes. This can be as efficient monaurally as binaurally. The echoes result from reflections of sound within the pinna; sound arriving from above will produce an echo faster than that from below, at about 100 and 300 microseconds respectively.

Horizontal localization is mainly a function of balanced binaural hearing and is due to:

- The head shadow effect. This arises when short wavelength sound, that is the higher frequencies above approximately 1500 Hz, are attenuated by reflection off the head. An average intensity difference of about 6 dB occurs between the two ears in this way. The longer wavelength lower frequencies tend to bend around the head (diffract) so are not attenuated significantly.
- Difference in time of arrival. This has an effect on the lower frequencies, which bend around the head to reach the opposite ear. A difference of about 600 milliseconds will arise between the ears.

- Phase difference. This only affects sound below 1500 Hz as the wavelength must be greater than the distance between the ears.

(b) The external auditory meatus

The ear canal has two main functions. Firstly, it is involved in protection; the cerumen and hairs along its outer lining help to protect the ear from foreign bodies and to prevent dirt from reaching the tympanic membrane; also, being curved, it can protect the drum and middle ear from trauma. Secondly, the canal acts as a resonance tube. The average canal is about 2.5 cm long, and at this length the resonant frequency lies at about 3 kHz. Sound around this frequency is amplified, usually by about 10 dB to 15 dB, although wide inter-individual variations do occur.

(c) The middle ear

Once the sound has reached the tympanic membrane, the alternating compressions and rarefactions of the sound wave move the drum in and out, and with it the handle of the malleus. The actual movement of the drum is quite complex and varies with different frequencies. The incus moves with the malleus, rocking on a linear axis running through the neck of the malleus and the body and short process of the incus. These movements are transmitted to the stapes, which also has a complex mode of movement, sometimes in and out as a piston or more of a rocking action; this, too, is frequency and intensity dependent.

The function of the middle ear is to conduct sound to the cochlea efficiently. In order to do this it must overcome the impedance mismatch between air and the cochlear fluids. It takes considerably more force to disturb fluid molecules than those of air, and the middle ear acts as a transformer to build up the pressure to a sufficient level. The overall gain is between 25 dB and 30 dB. This is achieved in several ways:

- Areal ratio. The tympanic membrane has a much larger area than the oval window, 65 mm^2 and 3.2 mm^2 respectively, which represents a ratio of 20:1. The effective area of the drum, that is excluding the pars flaccida, is about two-thirds of the total, giving an actual ratio of about 15:1. The force is therefore concentrated on to a much smaller area.
- Leverage action. Due to the relative position of the ossicles, the malleus and incus tend to move together as a single unit with the effective fulcrum lying nearer to the stapes. This produces an increase in leverage at the stapes footplate of 1.32:1.
- Characteristics of the tympanic membrane itself. The conical shape of the drum tends to concentrate sound energy, particularly high

frequencies, at the umbo. As the drum is set at an oblique angle in the meatus, this effectively increases the surface area. These contributions are fairly minimal.

The two muscles of the middle ear, the stapedius and the tensor tympani, have an important role to play in the conductive function of the middle ear. They produce an increase in the impedance of the ossicular chain by introducing stiffness into the system. The overall acoustic impedance of the middle ear is dependent on both resistance, or friction, which is independent of frequency, and reactance, a combination of stiffness and mass, which is frequency-dependent. A system with high reactance due to stiffness will impede the lower frequencies far more than the higher frequencies.

The more important of the two muscles is the stapedius. On contraction, this pulls backwards and slightly outwards, thus reducing movement of the stapes in the oval window. This is most effective for lower frequency sounds. In normally-hearing ears, pure tone stimuli between the range 70 dB to 90 dB above threshold will cause the muscle to contract in both the ipsilateral and the contralateral ear; the level may be lower for noise. The predictable nature of this response, the stapedial reflex, is used diagnostically (section 12.2.7). More reliable contraction is obtained below 250 Hz and attenuation here can be in the order of 20 dB to 30 dB. Above 1000 Hz it becomes unreliable, producing minimal attenuation.

The tensor tympani contracts as part of the overall 'startle' response. The muscle requires sound at high intensity to produce contraction, which then pulls forwards and slightly inwards, tensing the drum and producing more reflection of sound. The tensor tympani will also contract following tactile stimuli, such as puffing air on the cornea, or touching the meatus. It is less predictable than the stapedial reflex, but at high sound levels it is difficult to separate the two responses.

The reflexes serve to protect the ear from high intensity sound. However, this is ineffective with very transient noise, such as gunfire, as there is a delay in muscle contraction. There is certainly a function in protecting the ears from continuous acoustic trauma and from one's own voice when shouting. The reflex is also thought to improve speech intelligibility in noise, as the higher frequencies are attenuated less and the masking effect is thus reduced.

Most conduction of sound to the inner ear is by the route described, across the middle ear; this is called air conduction. Some sound energy, however, is transmitted directly to the cochlea through the bones of the skull, bypassing the middle ear. This fact is used clinically to assess the ability of the inner ear to hear sound without any interference from the outer or middle ear functions. Bone conduction is one of the normal routes of hearing for some sound, particularly of one's own voice. The cochlea is stimulated by bone conduction in three ways:

- By direct stimulation from vibrations of the skull. The round window is less rigid than the oval window, so pressure release is possible; this is the compression effect.
- By vibration of the ossicular chain, hence the reduction in bone conduction thresholds with ossicular fixation, such as otosclerosis (Carhart's notch). This is known as the inertial effect.
- From sound radiating into the meatus and producing pseudo-air conduction. This is linked with the occlusion effect, where occlusion of the meatus produces an enhancement of low frequency sound within the meatus, together with a reduction in masking by ambient noise.

Malformation, damage or disease in any part of the conduction apparatus produces a conductive hearing loss.

2.2.2 THE PERCEPTION OF SOUND

The apparatus for perception of sound is the sense-organ of hearing, the organ of Corti, contained in the cochlea. Here sound is first analysed into its component frequencies before being relayed to the auditory areas of the brain via the cochlear nerve.

Cochlear function can be thought of as two essential processes, transmission and transduction. Transmission is the transference of acoustic energy from the oval window to the organ of Corti. Transduction is the means by which this sound energy is converted to electrical impulses in the auditory nerve fibres.

(a) The transmission process

The theories of von Békèsy, first described in 1943, still form the basis of our understanding of this process. His 'travelling wave theory' describes how vibrations at the oval window of a frequency greater than 20 Hz, set up a wave along the basilar membrane, beginning at the base of the cochlea and travelling towards the apex. At some point, this wave attains a maximum displacement. Where the peak displacement of the wave arises is dependent on the frequency of the sound and how its passage is impeded by the varying mass and stiffness of the membrane. Lower frequencies pass further along the membrane and reach a peak nearer the apex, whereas the peak for high frequencies lies nearer the base. The position of the peak is very highly tuned and is determined very precisely by the frequency of the stimulating sound (Figure 2.11).

This tuning of the basilar membrane is important for frequency

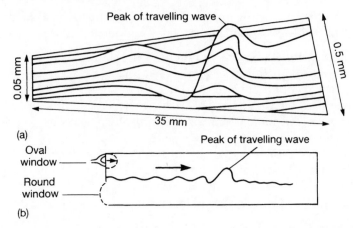

Fig. 2.11 Békèsy's travelling wave concept: the movement of the stapes in the oval window creates a travelling wave (a), which moves along the basilar membrane. Pressure is released via the round window (b).

discrimination, although later experiments have shown that tuning is even more precise, involving individual groups of hair cells, and it appears that the cochlea is not a purely passive structure. The outer hair cells, activated by efferent nerve fibres, are thought to play a part in selectively stiffening the basilar membrane, thus sharpening its response by 'vibration amplification'. Otoacoustic emissions or 'cochlear echoes', which are by-products of the outer hair cells' contribution to vibration, can be measured in the ear canal. Otoacoustic emissions are linked to hearing ability and are currently used to provide an objective method of screening hearing in babies. For low intensity sound the hair cells are stimulated by individual frequencies. As the sound pressure level rises, there is a larger displacement of the membrane with more groups of hair cells being stimulated, and the fine tuning is thus reduced. Other mechanisms are then involved further along the auditory pathway, which increases the accuracy of information reaching the auditory cortex.

(b) The transduction process within the cochlea

The tectorial membrane does not move in the same way as the basilar membrane; when the wave travels along it causes the tectorial membrane to move forwards as well as upwards, then backwards as well as downwards. The stereocilia of the hair cells are embedded in the tectorial membrane and this shearing motion bends them first one way, towards the tallest stereocilia, and then the other way, away from it. Joining their tips are 'transduction links' (Figure 2.12) and the tension on these is alternately tightened and released. Normally in the resting

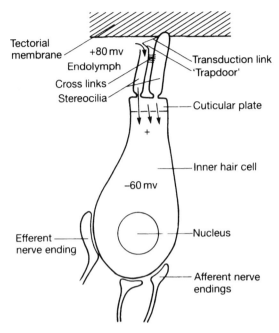

Fig. 2.12 The transduction links between the stereocilia of a hair cell. (An inner hair cell is shown.) Shearing of the stereocilia is thought to cause a 'trap door' to open at the top of each stereocilium and the intracellular potential is driven more positive.

position the endolymph outside the hair cell has a positive charge of approximately 80 millivolts, while the inside of the cell has a negative charge of approximately −60 millivolts. It is thought that as the transduction links tighten a 'trap door' opens at the top of each cilia. An electrical potential gradient is thus set up, which causes an ionic intercharge and results in the hair cell becoming more positively charged. This, in turn, stimulates release of neurotransmitters at the base of the cell, which fire the nerve impulse; a wave of depolarization passes down the length of the axon. This nerve impulse is called the action potential and can be recorded by placing electrodes in the cochlea. The value of the potential is a few millivolts and is fixed; that is, a higher intensity sound produces more firing of the action potentials but not larger potentials.

Other potentials have been found in the cochlea by using recording electrodes:

- The cochlear microphonic. This has a maximum value of 3–4 millivolts and is an alternating current (AC) potential, which arises in the outer hair cells in response to a sound stimulus. It is a voltage analogue of the original waveform, which remains linear to about 100 dBSPL and then saturates. It has proved valuable in research and also in assessing cochlear function in diagnostic investigation.

- Summating potential. This again arises from the outer hair cells. It is a direct current (DC) potential that is usually negative. It tends to occur in response to high intensities and is the sum of various responses to the travelling waveform envelope.

Understanding of the perception of sound is increasing with new research. Since the concept of von Békèsy was published there have been many refinements. It is now known that the nerve fibres themselves show frequency selectivity and that they have a spontaneous firing rate of just above 0–150 per second. Firing of the nerves occurs only at particular phases of the waveform, allowing a temporal regularity in response to a periodic stimulus. The fibres themselves are distributed in an orderly manner in the main auditory nerve bundle. Fibres that respond to high frequencies are on the periphery, graduating to those responding to the lowest frequencies right in the centre.

Malformation, damage or disease occurring in any part of the perceptive apparatus may cause sensorineural hearing loss.

(c) The central connections of the cochlear nerve

The nerve cells that supply the cochlea are described as bi-polar. That is they each have a body and two axons. One axon terminates at the base of a hair cell and the other in the cochlear nucleus of the brainstem. The cell bodies themselves are grouped together in the osseous spiral lamina of the cochlea and thus called the spiral ganglion. All groups of nerve cell bodies in the peripheral nervous system are called ganglia, whereas in the central nervous system they are called nuclei.

From the spiral ganglion, the nerve fibres join together to form the cochlear nerve and pass through the internal auditory canal, to enter the brainstem. From here the nerve divides into two and terminates in the ventral and dorsal cochlear nuclei. Most fibres from these nuclei cross over to the superior olivary nucleus of the opposite hemisphere. The pathway continues via the lateral lemniscus, the inferior colliculus, the medial geniculate body and then on to the auditory cortex. There is also crossing of fibres at the level of the inferior colliculus. Some fibres follow this pathway on the same side, thus the cortex of each hemisphere receives information from both ears, but the majority of information received in the left auditory cortex will have originated in the right ear (Figure 2.13).

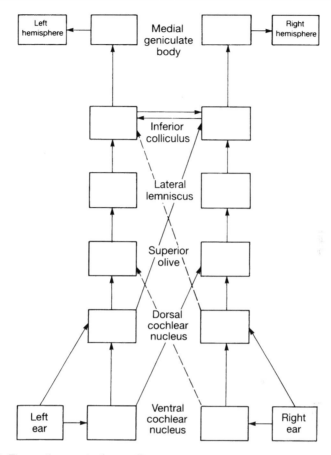

Fig. 2.13 The pathways to the auditory cortex.

2.3 SUMMARY

This chapter deals with the essential anatomical information required to understand the functioning of the human ear. Beginning with the only visible part of the ear, the pinna, it proceeds through each of the three parts: the external, middle and inner ear. Included are the essential relationships of the middle ear cavity, the complex anatomy of the cochlea and labyrinth and the organs of hearing and balance. Finally the chapter deals with the nasopharynx and the central connections of the cochlear nerve.

The current understanding of the function of the human ear in receiving and perceiving sound can be described under two headings:

- the conduction of sound – explaining how the conductive apparatus of the ear collects and transmits the sound from the air to the fluid of the inner ear;
- the perception of sound – how the inner ear and the sensory organ of hearing convert the sound energy into nerve impulses for relaying to the auditory cortex.

FURTHER READING

Ballantyne, D. (1990) *Handbook of Audiological Techniques*, Butterworth-Heinnemann, London, pp. 28–51.

McCormick, B. (1988) *Paediatric Audiology 0–5 years*, Taylor and Francis, London, pp. 221–46.

Pickles, J.O. (1982) *An Introduction to the Physiology of Hearing*, Academic Press, London.

von Békèsy, G. (1960) *Experiments in Hearing*, McGraw-Hill, New York.

Medical aspects of hearing loss

3

3.1 INTRODUCTION

Hearing loss may be due to a wide variety of pathological processes occuring in any part of the ear. 'Pathology' means the study of disease. Diseases, or disorders, can be considered under the following headings:

- traumatic, or from injury;
- infective, or from micro-organisms;
- tumours;
- iatrogenic, caused by physician or surgeon, by use of inappropriate medication, surgical accident or unsterile operation;
- idiopathic, or of unknown cause;
- physiological disorders, including degenerative effects of ageing;
- congenital, or from birth, whether inherited or caused by environmental factors.

Human cells contain 23 pairs of chromosomes. Twenty-two pairs are known as autosomes and are numbered 1 to 22. The remaining two chromosomes (one pair) are known as sex chromosomes. Abnormalities may involve the autosomes or the sex chromosomes, or they may involve only individual genes. All hereditary characteristics, for example eye colour, are carried by genes on the chromosomes.

Congenital defects may be due to 'environmental' factors (such as illness during pregnancy), but a high proportion of congenital deafness is inherited. In some inherited conditions the symptoms may not be apparent at birth, but may develop later in life. Many malformations or traits occur together and these may be termed as a syndrome. A family history will generally determine whether an inherited trait is dominant, recessive, or sex-linked.

3.2 PATHOLOGY OF THE OUTER EAR

3.2.1 CONGENITAL CONDITIONS OF THE OUTER EAR

(a) Malformation of the pinna

Sometimes children are born with an accessory, or extra, pinna, or a tag of soft tissue and cartilage. This may be large or quite small, and it may be situated away from the normal site of ear formation. Treatment is by removal. Both microtia (poorly developed pinna) and anotia (no pinna) may be associated with other abnormalities of the conductive auditory system and are therefore an indicator for further investigation.

(b) Aural fistula

An aural fistula or sinus may be present. This can be quite a deep channel leading from the skin surface. Deep removal may be necessary or it can become cystic. The operation must be very carefully done as the facial nerve runs past this area and damage can lead to facial paralysis and permanent disfigurement.

(c) Atresia

Atresia can be present, in which case there is complete closure, or absence, of the external auditory meatus, and an operation is required to make an opening. There may be a partial closure or extreme narrowness (stenosis) of the canal by an overgrowth of bone in or along the meatus, and this may go with a partial lack of development of the mid-face.

(d) Hereditary conditions

Hereditary conditions are those that are passed down to children from their parents due to genetic defects. There are a number of conditions that are hereditary and culminate in a lack of growth of parts of the face; probably the best example that affects the outer ear is Treacher Collin's syndrome. The main defects in this case may be poorly-formed cheek-bones, poorly-formed pinnae, sloping eyes with nicks in the eyelids (colobomas) and hearing impairment (see also section 3.3.1).

3.2.2 ACQUIRED CONDITIONS OF THE OUTER EAR

(a) Injury to the pinna

The pinna may be damaged by injury or trauma. The most common injury is a bruising or haematoma, which is a collection of blood in the tissues, often caused by boxing or an assault. Treatment should be carried out as early as possible, by aspirating away the blood with a syringe, or by making an incision to drain it. If this is not undertaken, the pressure of the contained blood can cause a local death of the tissues and formation of scar tissue, which may result in a 'cauliflower ear'.

Sometimes an earlobe is torn, often when wearing ear-rings. There may even be the complete loss of a pinna. If possible, any cartilage should be retained for later plastic surgery reconstruction. It is difficult to apply a plastic false ear to the side of the head securely, so either a loop of tissue is formed, or dental osseo-integrated implants are inserted into the mastoid bone to aid retention.

(b) Injury to the tympanic membrane

Most commonly this is caused by children poking objects into their own or other people's ears. It can also be caused by unskilled treatment or syringing, or by a slap or blow on the ear. Gunfire or explosion can cause even greater damage as the initial explosive pressure is followed by an air vacuum and suction.

In a similar way, the eardrum can be damaged by barotrauma, which is a rapid alteration in air pressure caused by the sudden descent of an unpressurised aircraft or rapid ascent from deep sea diving. The drum may also be involved when the temporal bone of the skull is fractured by a sideways blow, when a car is hit by an object side on, for example.

The symptoms are usually pain with minimal bleeding, deafness, tinnitus and vertigo. The signs are bleeding or a visible tear on the drum. It is best not to syringe or clear the ear but to give systemic antibiotics and leave it to heal.

(c) Foreign bodies

Objects in the ears are relatively common, especially in children. Hard objects, such as beads, can be hooked out. Soft objects of any sort, except vegetable matter, which can swell up when wetted, can all be syringed out, as shown in Figure 3.1. Forceps and tweezers are not generally used as these may push objects even further in, but a special loop can sometimes be used successfully. All such removals should be undertaken by a medically-qualified person.

Insects occasionally enter the ear and cause intense irritation by their buzzing. This can be deadened by pouring warm olive oil into the canal.

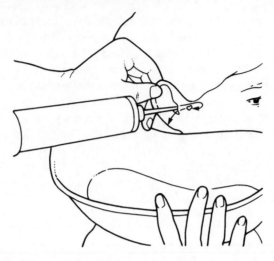

Fig. 3.1 Syringing the ear.

(d) Excessive wax

Wax may accumulate in the external auditory meatus. New wax is soft and moist, and light in colour. With age, wax becomes dark and hard. It may sometimes block the meatus and, if impacted, it may press on the drum. Excessive wax can disturb hearing.

Wax may be removed by syringing, often after it has been softened using drops of warmed olive oil, or similar, for a few days. Syringing should not be undertaken if there is any suspicion of a perforation, and otologists generally remove wax dry, often using a wax hook.

(e) Infection of the outer ear

Generally speaking, infections may be caused by all kinds of micro-organisms, bacteria, viruses, fungi, lice, worms and so on. Infection in the nasal passages and sinuses is controlled by the mucous cells lining these areas, which have myriads of small moving hair-like processes called cilia. These all act in unison to clear bacteria away. In the ears, bacteria and dust are extruded in the soft wax. In the mouth and throat, bacteria can be washed away in the saliva which itself has some antiseptic properties, as do the tears in the eyes.

The reaction of the tissues to infection is known as inflammation. The blood vessels enlarge, lymphocytes and macrophage cells collect in the area and migrate through the vessel walls to mop up the infective organisms (phagocytosis). Drainage of the infected area is via the lymphatic vessels to the relevant lymph nodes, which can become enlarged and tender.

Whether the inflammation controls the infection depends on the virulence of the organism, and also on the health and resistance of the individual. If the person is unfit, perhaps on a poor diet, anaemic or diabetic, resistance will be impaired and the infection could therefore worsen. Some bacteria give off toxins that lower the resistance of the tissues and facilitate the spread of the infection.

Viruses are smaller particles than bacteria and have no cell membrane of their own; they can only live and multiply in the cells of the host. Viruses do not respond to ordinary antibiotics. Treatment can be by antivirals and analgesics and by boosting the patient's general fitness.

Otitis externa, or acute dermatitis of the outer ear, is an inflammation of the skin covering the pinna or lining the external auditory meatus. The condition often occurs in conjunction with dandruff of the scalp. It can cause extreme irritation and scratching of the area, which may be due to staphylococcus, or to fungi, which collect in any cracks. This can be remedied by treating the dandruff and by local application of antibiotic creams or fungicides.

Eczema or sensitization dermatitis, is an allergic form of skin inflammation that can cause vesicles and oozing. (A vesicle is a small swelling filled with a clear exudate – not with pus.) The ear should be cleaned carefully and any general allergy should be treated.

Herpes is an infection with a particular virus of the herpes family. **Herpes simplex** may cause a bright red inflammation and ulceration, but usually heals within ten days. **Herpes zoster (shingles)** is a much more virulent type similar to the virus of chicken-pox. It causes an acute inflammation of the sensory nerve ganglions, and when this occurs in the auditory, facial and trigeminal nerves it causes vesicles and severe pain in the area of the face that is innervated by the particular nerve affected. The disease may continue for a long time and may recur despite treatments.

Furunculosis is the presence of a furuncle, or boil, which is caused by infection of the hair follicle by staphylococcus bacteria. Boils within the cartilage in the external auditory meatus are excruciatingly painful, and any swelling may cause a hearing loss. Treatment is with antibiotics and the application of warm glycerine and antiseptic on the area using a soft cotton wool wick in the ear passage.

Otomycosis is a fungal infection and is treated by keeping the ear dry and applying nystatin or other antifungal ointments.

(f) Tumours

Tumours may be either benign or malignant (cancerous).

Benign tumours are commonly exostoses, or outgrowths, of normal bone and are usually referred to as osteoma. These may be left alone if small but, if large and interfering with hearing, they can be removed with a small dental-type drill, using an operating microscope.

The most common malignant tumour in this area is the basal cell carcinoma, or rodent ulcer. This usually affects the upper edge of the pinna probably being brought on by ultraviolet sunlight. It may appear as an ulcer that fails to heal and, if left, it can spread to the scalp and inner ear, and cause great destruction of the tissues.

Malignant skin cancer can spread via the lymphatic scavenger system and can appear in the auricular or cervical lymph nodes. Early removal is made by cutting a V-shaped notch in the pinna including a 10 mm surround of healthy tissue to prevent recurrence. If left, it can involve the facial nerve and cause a facial palsy and unbearable pain. Any affected lymph nodes in the area of the neck must also be removed by an extensive operation.

3.3 PATHOLOGY OF THE MIDDLE EAR

3.3.1 CONGENITAL CONDITIONS OF THE MIDDLE EAR

In certain disorders, which are mainly hereditary genetic abnormalities, there may be a malformation of the middle ear, such as a lack of, or malformation of, one or more of the ossicles. Some examples include:

Treacher Collin's syndrome	Autosomal-dominant genetic defect, leading to poorly-formed cheek-bones, fish-like mouth, sloping eyes, nicks in the eyelids (colobomas), poorly-developed outer and middle ears, often with atresia of ear canals. Hearing defects are mainly conductive.
Crouzon's syndrome	Autosomal-dominant. Lack of growth mid-face, abnormally-shaped head with central prominence in the frontal region. Hearing defects that are mainly conductive.
Down's syndrome	Chromosomal abnormality (the presence of an extra number 21 chromosome), resulting in learning difficulties and classic facial features including small pinnae and narrow ear canals. High incidence, about 1 in 700 live births; risk increases with age of mother. Hearing defects may be conductive, sensorineural or mixed.

| Paget's disease | Autosomal-recessive skeletal disorder. Progressive deformities become apparent around the second year of life. Mixed progressive hearing loss due to continued new bone formation at base of skull. |

3.3.2 ACQUIRED CONDITIONS OF THE MIDDLE EAR

(a) Traumatic conditions

Trauma may be direct – for example, damage caused by poking an object into the middle ear – or it may be indirect, often due to a blow on the side of the head, which may cause damage to the temporal bone. Symptoms of the latter are usually bleeding from the ear, bruising over the mastoid bone, pain and deafness. Signs may include a split in the tympanic membrane, haemorrhage in the ear canal, facial palsy and other signs of local nerve damage. Radiographically there may be signs of fracture in the temporal area, which is confirmed by a computerized tomogram (CT) scan. Treatment is by cleaning the ear canal, and giving antibiotics systemically. Syringing should not be undertaken.

(b) Infective conditions

Otitis media   Otitis media is an inflammation of the middle ear, which is usually accompanied by some temporary loss of hearing.

Air enters the Eustachian tube during swallowing in order to balance the air pressure in the middle ear with ambient atmospheric pressure. If the Eustachian tube is blocked, which is often due to infection, normal middle ear pressure cannot be maintained because oxygen is absorbed by the tissues. The resultant negative pressure causes fluid to exude from the walls of the middle ear. The fluid may be sterile or infected (pus) and it may build up sufficiently to cause painful pressure on the eardrum. If the eardrum bursts, the fluid is released, the pain subsides, and the Eustachian tube gradually clears and opens again. A perforation in the lower part of the eardrum is considered safe and will usually heal uneventfully, although it may leave an area of weakened scar tissue. A perforation in the upper part of the eardrum is considered dangerous because of its close proximity to important structures. Middle ear infection is treated by antibiotics and painkillers.

Children are very prone to otitis media because their Eustachian tubes are more horizontal than those of adults and their immune systems are less well developed. Where the condition is recurrent, a

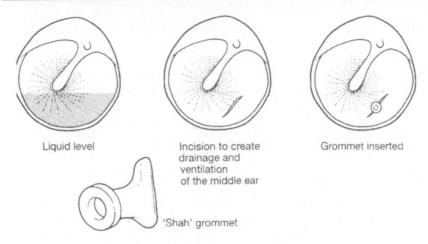

Liquid level

Incision to create
drainage and
ventilation
of the middle ear

Grommet inserted

'Shah' grommet

Fig. 3.2 'Glue ear' – secretory otitis media and its treatment.

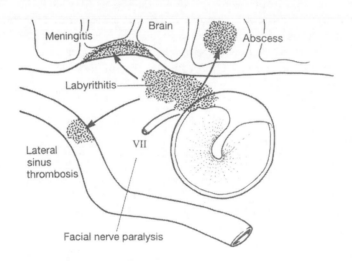

Meningitis

Brain

Abscess

Labyrithitis

Lateral
sinus
thrombosis

VII

Facial nerve paralysis

Fig. 3.3 Otitis media with complications.

sticky residue may adhere to the ossicles, inhibiting their movement
and causing a hearing loss. This condition is commonly known as 'glue
ear'. Where otitis media is long-standing or repeated, or in cases of
glue ear, a myringotomy may be undertaken. A small incision is made
in the lower part of the drum to release the fluid and a plastic grommet
may be inserted in the eardrum (Figure 3.2) to ventilate the middle ear
and thus prevent recurrence.

If not treated early enough, middle ear infection may spread and
can result in major dangerous disease, such as meningitis or a brain
abscess (Figure 3.3), symptoms being acute headache and very high

temperature. Before the use of antibiotics, middle ear infection often caused an infection of the mastoid air cells (mastoiditis) and the best cure at that time was a mastoidectomy, which was a painful and dangerous operation to open up and drain the area. Early recognition and treatment with antibiotics is therefore of great importance and may be life-saving.

Cholesteatoma Dangerous chronic (long-standing) otitis media usually occurs in a middle ear where the Eustachian tube is never fully open. The air pressure is lower in the middle ear than in the external ear canal, thus the greater external air pressure gradually pushes into the soft, flaccid upper part of the drum to form a pouch. Epithelial skin cells lining the ear canal are continually being shed and migrate naturally out of the ear canal, but those within this pouch cannot be cleared away by natural migration. Gradually an accumulation of skin cells, wax, dust and bacteria builds up into a sticky mass which is termed a cholesteatoma. This builds up further, becomes more infected, pushes into the outer attic wall (Figure 3.4) and begins to discharge a foul-smelling pus. As it enlarges further it can destroy the ossicular chain and may even erode the roof of the middle ear and cause intracranial infections. It may also burst through and damage the labyrinth and/or the facial nerve to cause a facial palsy. Symptoms and signs are of a recurrent foul discharge, pain, deafness and possibly vertigo. Treatment is by operating, opening the area widely and cleaning the whole middle ear and mastoid air cells, cleaning out the cholesteatoma and drying up any discharge. If untreated, the complications can be very serious indeed.

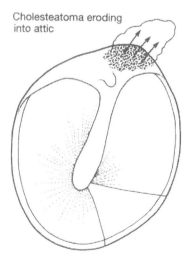

Cholesteatoma eroding into attic

Fig. 3.4 Cholesteatoma following chronic suppurative otitis media.

(c) Facial paralysis

Facial paralysis may arise from damage to the facial nerve via the mastoid air cells (Figure 2.7), or the nerve may be damaged in an accident or operation. Paralysis of the muscles of facial expression results, causing marked asymmetry of the face, with possible loss of taste and salivation. People thus affected cannot smile, raise their eyebrows or close the eye of the affected side. If long term, the eyelids may have to be sewn together to protect the eye. If the cause is unknown, it is termed a Bell's palsy. Treatment is often with steroids. There is also a surgical procedure, called facial hypoglossal anastomosis, to re-route the facial nerve. In addition, these patients may be referred to a physiotherapist or speech and language therapist for facial exercises and/or electrical or thermal stimulation.

(d) Otosclerosis

Otosclerosis is an exuberant growth of normal bone, the cause of which is unknown. It usually affects the middle ear but may also affect the inner ear. Extra spongy-type bone is produced, especially around the oval and round windows. This spongy bone gradually hardens. The stapes may therefore become immoveable causing deafness. The condition occurs in young adults and there may be a family history. It may be accelerated during pregnancy, probably due to hormonal activity.

A conductive hearing loss will be present, which is greatest in the low frequencies. A dip in the bone conduction threshold at 2 kHz is often noted (Figure 3.5 (a)). This is known as Carhart's notch. In later stages of otosclerosis, there may be sensorineural involvement as the bony growth invades the inner ear. Treatment is by microscopic surgery, the stapes being removed wholly or partly and replaced with a prosthesis, which may be a small metal or Teflon plunger wedged into place at the oval window with a piece of foam or fat (Figure 3.6). The operation is all done through an incision in the tympanic membrane, and the working end of the piston is usually hooked around the bottom end of the incus. The operation is termed a stapedectomy.

3.4 PATHOLOGY OF THE INNER EAR

In the inner ear, disease may produce dizziness due to a disturbance of fluid levels in the labyrinth, or it may affect the cochlea or the auditory nerve causing sensorineural hearing loss. As before, diseases may be classified as congenital or acquired.

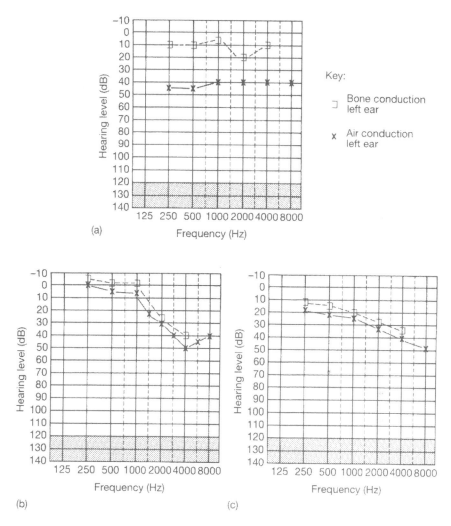

Key:

⊐ Bone conduction
   left ear

x Air conduction
   left ear

(a)

(b)

(c)

Fig. 3.5 Audiograms for the left ear illustrating (a) otosclerosis, (b) typical noise damage, (c) presbyacusis.

3.4.1 CONGENITAL CONDITIONS OF THE INNER EAR

Congenital hearing loss may be caused by maldevelopment of the inner ear, as in hereditary genetic abnormalities, or by environmental damage such as occurs when infectious diseases in the mother cross over the placenta to affect the unborn child, for example, syphilis, CMV and German measles (rubella). Development can also be affected by severe jaundice, such as that due to rhesus factor antibodies in the

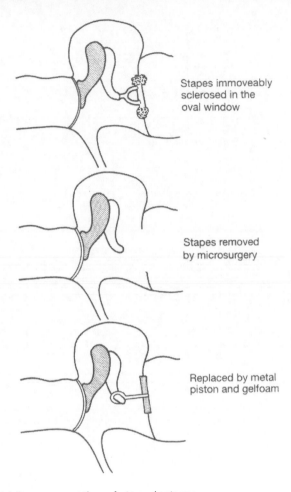

Stapes immoveably sclerosed in the oval window

Stapes removed by microsurgery

Replaced by metal piston and gelfoam

Fig. 3.6 The middle-ear operation of stapedectomy.

mother's blood, or by other neonatal/perinatal factors such as anoxia, or use of antibiotic drugs. Many congenital hearing losses of unknown cause are thought to be non-syndromic genetic losses. Examples of congenital conditions associated with sensorineural hearing loss include:

Usher's syndrome	Autosomal-recessive genetic condition. Moderate to severe bilateral sensorineural hearing loss is present at birth. Progressive blindness usually starts in teens due to retinitis pigmentosa.

Waardenburg's syndrome	Autosomal-dominant genetic condition. Features include white forelock, different coloured segments in the eyes and mild to profound hearing loss, which may be unilateral or bilateral, and sometimes progressive.
Turner's syndrome	Sex chromosome defect which is not inherited. Features include low hair-line, webbed neck, short stature, kidney defects and mild sensorineural and conductive hearing loss. Occurs only in females.
Rubella (German measles)	Viral infection contracted from the mother during pregnancy. Defects vary depending on the stage of development of the embryo/foetus when the infection occurs. Features include hearing loss, heart disease, eye disorders, psychomotor problems and behavioural disorders.
Cytomegalovirus disease (CMV)	Viral infection contracted from the mother during pregnancy or during birth. The disease in the mother may present very mild symptoms, such as a runny nose. In the baby, CMV affects the nervous system. Possible defects include hearing loss, learning difficulties, spasticity, convulsions and hyperactivity.
Syphilis	Bacterial infection contracted from the mother during pregnancy. Defects include slow progressive deafness and other sensory defects.

3.4.2 ACQUIRED CONDITIONS OF THE INNER EAR

Acquired inner ear diseases are those caused after birth, possibly by infection from mumps or meningitis, or they may be caused by an accident, blow or explosion, or by exposure to loud noise.

(a) Noise damage

Noise-induced hearing loss (NIHL) is caused by long exposure to high levels of noise, such as those found in certain industrial situations, especially prior to the *Noise at Work* regulations (Health and Safety Executive, 1989).

At first the noise will cause a temporary threshold shift (TTS), which is followed by full recovery after a period away from the noise, but after years of exposure the damage becomes permanent. The longer the duration and the more intense the noise, the greater will be the damage. Ear protection should be used and is now required by law above certain levels.

The greatest effect on hearing is in the high frequency region. The audiogram often shows a 'notch' at 4 kHz (Figure 3.5(b)), and the hearing loss is frequently accompanied by tinnitus.

Acoustic trauma is caused by intense short-duration sound, such as gunfire, and results in a sudden high frequency hearing loss.

(b) Presbyacusis and circulatory disorders

Presbyacusis is the term given to degeneration of hearing in old age. This is the most common general cause of hearing loss and results in a progressive bilateral sensorineural hearing loss, mainly in the high frequencies (Figure 3.5(c)). Presbyacusis can be thought of as the cumulative effect of living, and may include a variety of causes, such as:

- circulatory disorders, including arteriosclerosis, thrombosis and vascular spasm;
- noise damage, including long exposure at normal levels;
- poor diet;
- normal use of drugs;
- lack of exercise;
- stress.

Circulatory disorders are the most common specific cause of hearing loss. The cochlea requires a constant, sufficient supply of oxygen and nutrients to maintain its function. This supply is dependent on the condition of the heart, the blood vessels and the stria vascularis. Degenerative changes in the blood vessels, blood clots, high or low blood pressure, and damage due to elevated blood glucose levels in diabetes, may all affect hearing. Even a brief interruption to the blood supply may cause permanent damage.

(c) Infections

Infections affecting the inner ear are mainly viral or bacterial, although they may be due to other micro-organisms (section 3.2.2(e)).

Viral infections include:

- Mumps and measles may cause a sensorineural loss. The hearing loss caused by mumps is often unilateral. Measles may be complicated by otitis media.

- Shingles (herpes zoster) causes inflammation of the nerves and, if this involves the auditory nerve, will cause sensorineural loss with pain.
- Influenza can affect the cochlea via the bloodstream, often with an additional temporary conductive loss due to otitis media.

Bacterial infections include:

- Diphtheria may cause a sensorineural loss with secondary otitis media.
- Meningitis may cause sensorineural loss, which can be total. The meninges, or brain lining, is inflamed due to direct infection or neglected otitis media. The condition can be life-threatening and is usually treated with antibiotics. Some cases of meningitis are of viral origin.

Infections from the inner ear must be diagnosed and treated early because there can be a very dangerous spread of infection to the middle cranial fossa causing meningitis or a brain abscess, or the infection may spread into the neighbouring mastoid air cells, or infect the facial nerve to cause a palsy. Early treatment with antibiotics and surgical drainage may be life saving.

(d) Ototoxic drugs

Hearing loss due to drugs is usually bilateral, may be sudden or progressive, and is often accompanied by tinnitus. Some losses tend to recover (unless the dosage is very high) when the drug is withdrawn. For example, analgesics, such as aspirin, cause a reversible high frequency loss; diuretics, such as frusemide, cause a reversible low to mid frequency loss; and quinine causes a reversible low frequency loss. Other drugs, such as the powerful antibiotic streptomycin, cause permanent damage. Ototoxic drugs include:

streptomycin	quinine
aspirin	neomycin
chloramphenicol	frusemide
mercury	nitrogen mustard
kanamycin	gentamicin
chloroquine	thalidomide

(e) Conditions involving vertigo

Vertigo may occur in a number of conditions, most commonly through blockage of the Eustachian tube, suppuration in the labyrinth, tumours affecting the VIII cranial nerve, after operations on the ear and when affected by Menière's disorder.

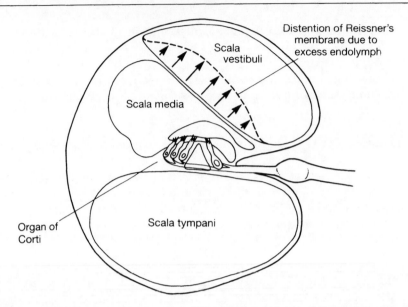

Fig. 3.7 Cross-section of the cochlea, to show expansion of the endolymphatic compartment in Menière's disorder and vestibular neuronitis.

Vertigo may be accompanied by nausea and vomiting, and nystagmus or vibrating movements of the eyes. Assessment will involve investigation of auditory and vestibular function. Tests usually include noting spontaneous and induced nystagmus, which provides valuable diagnostic information.

Menière's disorder, also known as idiopathic episodic endolymphatic hydrops, usually occurs in middle age. It is idiopathic as the cause is unknown, but it is known to be associated with a raised pressure on, and distension of, the membranous labyrinth (hydrops) (Figure 3.7). Symptoms are recurrent sudden attacks of dizziness, tinnitus and deafness. Nystagmus may also be present, and attacks may be nocturnal. The hearing loss is sensorineural, fluctuating. It is usually low frequency and may be unilateral. The condition must be referred for medical care. Hearing aids should only be recommended with the doctor's consent, as amplification can induce attacks.

Treatment is usually by medication with anti-sickness and antidepressant drugs. Alternative treatment can be by surgical decompression or destruction of the labyrinth with an ultrasonic beam or a laser. Surgical destruction may stop the symptoms but deafness thereafter will be complete. Other treatment includes reduction of fluid, restricting salt in the diet and prescribing diuretics, which increase fluid excretion.

Vestibular neuronitis is a condition similar to Menière's disorder, but the cause, a virus, is known, and it normally affects younger people.

Acoustic neuroma is a benign (local, slow-growing) tumour, or neuro-fibroma, of the VIII cranial nerve. The condition is relatively rare, having an incidence of 1 in 100 000 population (O'Donoghue, 1993), but may be fatal if it is not surgically treated. Its symptoms may be similar to Menière's disorder, and clinical assessment includes tests (described in Chapter 12) to distinguish these conditions. Diagnosis is usually by a CT scan, and treatment is by neurosurgery. An acoustic neuroma is actually an overgrowth of the Schwann cells of the outer sheath of the nerve trunk, and has to be approached by drilling a hole in the skull.

Other causes of vertigo with hearing loss can be:

• postural after head injuries;
• impaired blood supply to the brain;
• infections such as syphilis;
• tumours such as cancer;
• obstructed Eustachian tubes;
• build up of wax causing pressure;
• the taking of ototoxic drugs.

3.5 OTHER CONDITIONS OF THE EAR

3.5.1 OPERATIONS ON THE EAR

Myringotomy is an operation for treating secretory otitis media (glue ear), carried out under general anaesthetic, and in which a curved incision is made low down in the drum using a tiny, long-handled myringotomy knife. A Teflon drain or grommet may be put into the incision to keep the drain-hole open and thus provide ventilation (Figure 3.2). This grommet will normally be shed naturally within six months. If symptoms recur, the operation is repeated.

A **cortical mastoidectomy** is not used as often since the advent of powerful antibiotics. A curved incision is made behind the ear down to the mastoid process. The mastoid air cells and antrum are removed with bone drills and the cavity is left to drain. Great care must be taken to avoid damage to the facial nerve.

A **radical mastoidectomy** is undertaken in dangerous chronic disease. In this case, the entire mastoid and middle ear are drilled away including the malleus and incus. The base of the stapes is left sealing the oval window. The wound is protected with a gauze pad until the infection is controlled and then the area is grafted over with skin.

Tympanoplasty is reconstructive surgery performed under an operating microscope to replace the ossicles and to repair a torn or missing tympanic membrane.

Stapedectomy is an operation undertaken using an operating microscope; the eardrum is removed to provide access to the ossicles. The stapes is broken off the oval window and an artificial stapes is inserted. This may be a stainless steel or Teflon piston held in place by a fat graft or foam pad. The other end of the piston is hooked on to the incus. The drum is then replaced and packed with a sterile dressing to keep it in place for 48 hours, after which time the dressing is carefully removed. Results are normally very good.

Labyrinthectomy is usually undertaken to treat Menière's disorder or intractable tinnitus or vertigo. The mastoid and horizontal semicircular canal are drilled open so that the membranous labyrinth can be picked up and destroyed. As the middle ear is not opened in this operation healing should be quite quick, but hearing loss will be permanent.

All these operations have a much greater success rate since the advent of suitable antibiotics and with the use of operating microscopes and microsurgical techniques.

3.5.2. PAIN IN THE EAR

Otalgia or pain in the ear may be of local cause or referred from other areas.

(a) Local pain

The common local causes of earache are:

- boils in the external auditory meatus (these are especially painful in the cartilage; they are caused by an infection in a hair follicle by staphylococcus bacteria);
- otitis media, infection of the middle ear;
- mastoiditis, infection of the mastoid air cells;
- malignant disease of the ear.

(b) Referred pain

Pain may be referred from:

- decayed and infected molar teeth;
- impacted wisdom teeth;
- sinusitis, particularly from the maxillary sinus;
- herpes zoster (shingles), viral infection of the nerves;
- neck lesions, such as trapped cervical nerves;
- quinsy or tonsillar abscess;
- tongue with posterior ulcers or cancer;

- ulcers and cancers of the pharynx, larynx and palate;
- glossopharyngeal neuralgia (this is extremely painful);
- tempero-mandibular joint dysfunction;
- temporal arteritis;
- malignant diseased areas in close proximity to the ear.

Tempero-mandibular joint dysfunction is also known as Costen's syndrome. In this disease, pain from the joint arises from a malfunction due to damage, malformation, poor dental occlusion, loss of teeth or over-closure. Cases should be referred to an oral surgeon.

Temporal arteritis occurs when the outer wall of the temporal artery becomes diseased. The artery is swollen and painful to touch. A biopsy is taken and steroids prescribed or surgery advised.

Malignant diseases of the neighbouring areas, in particular the naso-pharynx, the back of the tongue, the palate or the floor of the mouth, may cause referred pain. A biopsy is required to confirm the diagnosis, followed by radiotherapy, chemotherapy, surgery or a combination thereof. Diagnosis must be early or the prognosis is very poor.

3.5.3 CONDITIONS INVOLVING TINNITUS

In these cases the clients complain of noises in the ear or head, possibly of pulsation, ringing, hissing or buzzing, usually associated with some loss of hearing.

Any abnormal condition of the ear can bring this on but the main causes are:

- otosclerosis – overgrowth of bone;
- wax secretions;
- tumours, benign and malignant;
- Menière's disorder;
- fevers;
- raised blood pressure (pulsating tinnitus);
- anaemia;
- nervous diseases (multiple sclerosis);
- taking of drugs and alcohol;
- over-smoking.

Surgery is not usually required, treatment being with sedatives, psychotherapy, kindness and care. For further information see section 12.1.

3.6 SUMMARY

Hearing loss may be conductive or sensorineural in type, or a mixture of these two.

Conductive hearing loss is caused by some abnormality of the outer or middle ear. The principal causes are:

- impacted wax blocking the ear canal;
- otitis externa or inflammation of the outer ear;
- otitis media or inflammation of the middle ear, glue ear if chronic;
- otosclerosis;
- atresia or stenosis;
- foreign bodies in the ear canal.

Treatment of any condition of the ears should only be undertaken by, or under the direction of, a medically-qualified person.

Sensorineural hearing loss is caused by some abnormality of the cochlea, auditory nerve or the hearing centres of the brain. Most sensorineural hearing loss is caused by defects or damage to the cochlea, due to:

- presbyacusis or the effects of age;
- vascular causes;
- excessive noise;
- hydrops or excessive fluid pressure in the inner ear;
- ototoxic drugs;
- congenital, hereditary and 'environmental' causes.

REFERENCES

Health and Safety Executive (1989) *Noise at Work*, HMSO, London.
O'Donoghue, G.M. (1993) Acoustic Neuroma: Triumph and Disaster. *British Journal of Hospital Medicine*, **49**(2), 86–7.

FURTHER READING

Birrell, J.F. (1982) *Logan Turner's Diseases of the Nose, Throat and Ear*, John Wright and Sons Ltd, Bristol.
Bull, P.D. (1981) *Lecture Notes on Diseases of the Ear, Nose and Throat*, Blackwell Scientific Publications, Oxford.
Ludman, H. (1988) *ABC of Ear, Nose and Throat*, British Medical Association, London.
Simson Hall, I. and Colman, B.H. (1987) *Diseases of the Nose, Throat and Ear*, 13th edn, Churchill Livingstone, Edinburgh.

Speech and intelligibility

4

4.1 THE SPEECH CHAIN

Speech is a most efficient means of communication that is resilient to background noise, interference and distortion. It can be understood despite different voices and accents, even on the telephone with no visual cues and a very restricted frequency range.

When most people consider speech, they think only of the lip and tongue movements and the sounds that they link with them; but speech is much more than just the act of speaking. It is concerned with both the production and the reception of spoken messages.

The speaker must decide what he wants to say, and form it into words and sentences according to the rules of English. He must then send impulses via his nervous system to the vocal organs to produce the speech sounds that travel through the air to the listener. The listener's ear receives the sounds and passes the messages to the brain, where they are finally decoded. Speech is a chain of events linking the speaker and the listener and is often called the speech chain (Figure 4.1).

The study of speech, which is known as phonetics, can be broken down into three main parts:

- articulatory phonetics is concerned with speech production;
- acoustic phonetics is concerned with the waveform, which provides the link between the speaker and the listener;
- auditory or perceptual phonetics is concerned with listening skills.

Written language is made up of a series of symbols or letters joined together to form words. These words are both formed and used according to certain rules, which are learned in early school and which

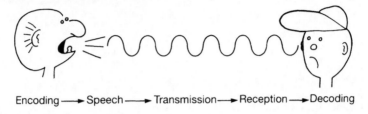

Encoding ——► Speech ——► Transmission ——► Reception ——► Decoding

Fig. 4.1 The speech chain.

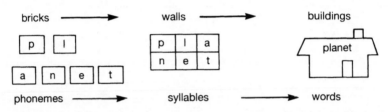

Fig. 4.2 The 'building bricks' that make up words.

later can be used with ease. Similarly, speech is made up of a series of sounds, which are formed into words. The individual sounds are called phonemes and these are the smallest units of sound that carry meaning; for example, the words c-a-t, c-o-t, c-u-t, are all made up of three phonemes. In each of these words, it is the medial phoneme which alters the meaning.

Phonemes are not identical to written letters, although there is much overlap. There are very approximately 40 phonemes in English, 20 vowels and 20 consonants, and an international phonetic alphabet (IPA) exists to symbolize these. Phonemes are built up into syllables; for example, planet is one word, but made up of two syllables and six phonemes. The phonemes can be likened to the bricks that build up into the walls (syllables), that are linked to make the buildings (words) (Figure 4.2).

In English, as in other languages, there are rules that constrain the way we build words from the individual sounds or phonemes, and we cannot use them in any order; for instance, 'klr' does not exist in English, while 'ng' only occurs at the end of a syllable, never at the beginning. Words, too, are joined together into sentences using certain rules of grammar (syntax) and meaning (semantics). Grammatical rules will tell us the order of words that is acceptable; for example, we know at once that 'Horse the I ride' is incorrect. However, grammar alone is not sufficient, as sentences must also make sense. 'The babysitting is high', for example, is meaningless, and so we can see that word order is constrained by both grammatical and semantic rules.

Most people could not state the rules of English but nevertheless rarely break them because they have an unconscious awareness of them.

4.2 THE VOCAL TRACT

The organs involved in speech production (Figure 4.3) are the lungs, trachea (windpipe), larynx (containing the vocal cords or folds), pharynx (throat), mouth and nose. The lungs produce the airstream, or power, to vibrate the vocal folds, which provide the source of sound. This is resonated by the vocal tract to produce recognizable speech sounds.

The airstream travels from the lungs up the trachea, through the larynx to the nose and mouth. The larynx acts as a valve between the throat and the lungs, able to open and close to control the airflow from the lungs. This action is largely dependent on the vocal cords, which are really folds of ligament, hence they are also known as the vocal folds. The space between the vocal folds is called the glottis, and when the vocal folds are open the glottis forms a 'V'-shape (Figure 4.4)

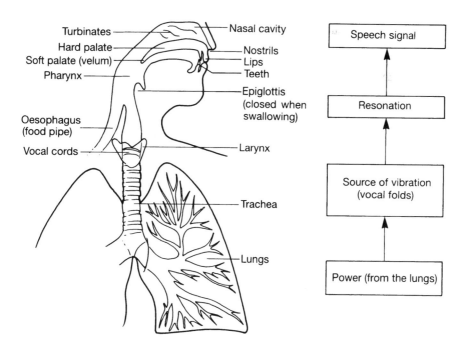

Fig. 4.3 The organs of the vocal tract and their role in the production of the speech signal.

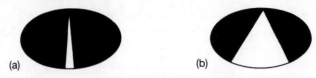

Fig. 4.4 Opening the vocal cords. (a) When lightly closed, the cords vibrate. (b) When spaced apart, the airflow is unimpeded.

because the vocal folds move away from each other only at the back of the trachea. As we speak, the air pressure from the lungs vibrates the vocal folds rhythmically. The frequency of the vibration depends upon how quickly the folds vibrate, and can be altered within a range of about an octave and a half.

The pharynx or throat connects the larynx with the mouth and nose. The nasal cavity extends from the pharynx and is divided by the septum into two sections leading to the nostrils. The walls of the two sections are not flat but have ridges and folds known as the turbinates. At the back of the nose and throat are the tonsils and adenoids. The nasal cavities can be closed off by raising the soft palate, in which case the airflow is directed through the mouth. The shape and size of the cavities of the mouth can be widely varied by moving the lips, teeth and tongue.

4.3 SPEECH-READING

The lips can be rounded, spread or closed, and in 'lip-reading' a deaf person watches the position of the lips and teeth to add information to the reduced sounds he or she hears. As well as watching the lip and teeth positions, most deaf people will also obtain other clues, or cues, from facial expression, posture, context and so on; this is often therefore called 'speech-reading'. Lip-reading is not sufficient alone because groups of sounds, known as visemes, look the same on the lips; for example 'p', 'b' and 'm' cannot be told apart by lip-reading. Discriminating individual sounds is made even more difficult in running speech, where the amount of lip-read information diminishes as we run one sound into another. Running speech is only easier to understand because other linguistic cues are present, not because of the lip-read patterns available.

When visual cues are combined with some hearing there can be very good speech perception; for example, lip-reading can disambiguate sentences that would sound the same, such as 'I'll have to see' and 'I'll have to sue'. These sentences can easily be differentiated by lip-reading.

Other linguistic cues are also important to comprehension, and language is rich in cues that we, as hearing people, do not often need to use. These cues are said to be redundant. Redundancy is present in all levels of language; for example, grammatical cues are signalled more than once in a sentence. The following sentences include a number of grammatical cues that signal plurality: 'This man is working', 'These men are working'.

Redundant cues are used as and when they are needed, for example, in background noise. High redundancy makes language very efficient because if we do miss parts, we can still understand the whole.

The hearing impaired cannot use all the cues available to the normally-hearing and evolve their own set, which is very individual. This is one reason why some hearing impaired people do so much better than others.

4.4 SPEECH SOUNDS

4.4.1 THE FORMATION OF VOWELS AND VOWEL-LIKE SOUNDS

The vocal tract is really a tube running from the lips at one end to the vocal cords (or vocal folds) at the other (Figure 4.3). A steady airstream, provided by the lungs, is set into vibration by the vocal cords, which are part of the larynx. The vocal cords open and close rapidly to create a sound, rather like a low frequency buzz, which is known as the fundamental laryngeal tone. This is the fundamental frequency of speech and it determines the pitch of the speaker's voice. The actual frequency or pitch is not fixed and depends on the rate of vibration of the vocal cords – the faster they vibrate, the more cycles per second and the higher the pitch. The average pitch is given in Table 4.1, but individuals can vary their voice pitch within a certain range.

Pure tones rarely occur in nature, and the sound source produced by vocal cord vibration contains nearly all possible harmonics. These reduce in intensity with increasing frequency, by about 12 dB per octave.

The vocal tract can be altered in shape by moving the lips, tongue and other articulators. The variation in shape modifies the sound spectrum by resonating some frequencies, thus increasing their amplitude, while damping, or reducing, others.

Table 4.1 The average frequency of vocal cord vibration

Subject	Frequency (Hz)
Man	120 Hz (B2)
Woman	220 Hz (A3)
Child	260 Hz (C4)

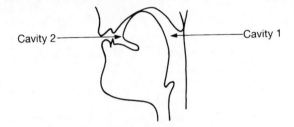

Fig. 4.5 The resonating cavities of the mouth.

When the neck of an empty bottle is blown across and then that of one partially filled with liquid, the changing column of air alters the resonant frequency and the resulting difference in pitch can be readily heard. The sound from the vocal cords is modified in a similar manner, especially by the mouth. The tongue effectively divides the vocal tract into two cavities – front and back (Figure 4.5), and the bigger the cavity, the lower is the resonant frequency produced.

The resonating cavities concentrate energy in particular frequency regions. These concentrations of energy into narrow bands are the basis of the vowel **formants**. The size and shape of the cavities determine the resonant frequencies, or formants. The vocal tract is highly variable and is changed primarily by the tongue and the lips. The first two formants are important in the recognition of vowels, the other formants are mainly used to distinguish who is speaking. Vowels are formed by altering the shape of the vocal tract without causing any constriction that would create friction, or aperiodic noise.

The vocal cord vibration is known as the fundamental frequency, which gives rise to the pitch of the voice. The shape of the vocal tract resonates the fundamental frequency, concentrating energy into narrow bands – formants. The fundamental frequency is not a formant.

Different speakers each produce slightly different sounds but we can interpret what we hear because the **relationship** between the formants remains unchanged. Each vowel can be likened to a chord in music, where the three notes played together can be recognized as a particular chord, no matter what key it is played in. Examples can be seen in Figure 4.6; the precise frequency values are not important.

All vowels contain the low frequency voicing, below 400 Hz, produced by the vocal cord vibration – the fundamental frequency – but they also have a formant structure, created by resonances of the vocal tract. The harmonics are still present but certain ones have been amplified by resonance into peaks of energy or formants, while others have been damped or filtered.

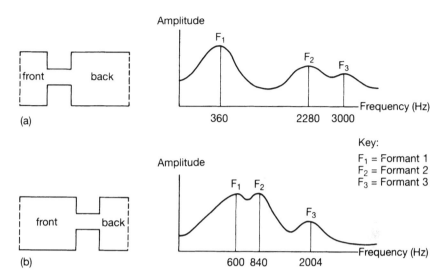

Fig. 4.6 The cavities of the mouth and the resultant formants of the vowels 'ee' (a) and 'aw' (b).

4.4.2 THE FORMATION OF APERIODIC CONSONANTS

Some consonants, such as the nasal consonants 'm', 'n' and 'ng', are vowel-like, but most consonants are aperiodic, that is they have a noise component. There are two methods by which these consonants can be produced.

1. The vocal tract is narrowed at some point so that the air has to push past, creating turbulence or friction. Consonants formed in this way are called **fricatives**. The waveform is irregular and aperiodic, that is it has a noise component. Some fricatives, such as 's', consist only of noise, others have a voiced component in addition, for example 'z'. It is often helpful to think of consonants in terms of voiced and voiceless pairs, for example:

Voiceless	Voiced
s	z
f	v

Voicing is a low frequency component caused by the vocal fold vibration.

2. The vocal tract is blocked at some point, such as at the lips, allowing the air pressure to build up, followed by a sudden release or plosion (Figure 4.7). These sounds are called **plosives**, for example 'p', and again they can be formed with or without accompanying vocal cord vibration (voicing), for example:

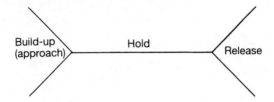

Fig. 4.7 The basic phases of a plosive.

Voiceless	Voiced
p	b
t	d

Consonants are usually described by the place and the manner in which they are formed. The important places of articulation in English are the lips, teeth, palate and glottis, although it is often sufficient to state the place of articulation as front, middle or back.

The manner of articulation may be plosive, fricative, nasal or 'semi-vowel'. Nasals and semi-vowels are produced without turbulence and closely resemble vowels. They are voiced and have a formant structure. Nasals are produced when the soft palate, or velum, is opened to permit airflow through the nose.

The complete description should include whether the sound is voiced or not, for example:

p can be described as a front voiceless plosive,
b can be described as a front voiced plosive,
f can be described as a front voiceless fricative.

4.4.3 UNDERSTANDING RUNNING SPEECH

In running speech, every sound is not formed carefully and precisely, but rather each individual sound is qualified by the sounds that come before and after. This requires less effort from the speaker, and in rapid speech a movement is often not finished but only started and then carried on towards the next. Speech is a continuum of rapid finely-skilled movements with much overlapping, of which the speaker is unaware but which is reflected in the acoustic spectrum.

Time is a very significant aspect of sound perception and the sounds of speech change continually. The formants of the vowels show some variation depending on the adjoining sounds. The articulators do not move instantaneously but rather 'glide' from one position to another. This can be observed on a spectrogram. The middle of the vowel, where the frequency is relatively stable, is called the **steady state**. The changing part is called the **transition** or glide. The transitions (Figure

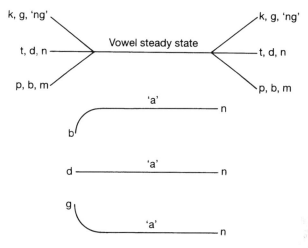

Fig. 4.8 Examples of transitions in the vowel formants.

4.8) are most obvious in formant two of the vowel, but are present to a lesser extent in other formants.

The transitions reflect the movement from one place of articulation to another. The noise of a consonant is normally the primary cue in recognition, but the transitions can be very important. Transitions exist in all formants but those in the second formant are the most important. However, it is likely that the hearing impaired may use the transitions in formant one, which are not important with normal hearing.

Time factors are also important in the recognition of speech and these can be carried at all levels of signal, so should be useful even to profoundly deaf people. In general, vowels are longer than consonants, although of course not all are the same length; some are very long and some relatively short, so, for example, 'ee' is about twice the length of 'i' ('ee' is approximately 285 milliseconds in length, 'i' is only approximately 147 milliseconds). Diphthongs are formed by the union of two vowel sounds and are therefore the longest of all vowel sounds. The length of a vowel is to some extent governed by the following consonant. A vowel will be longer if it is followed by a short consonant, and vice versa (Figure 4.9). These relative intensity cues are very important, especially to the hearing impaired.

Vowels have greater intensity than consonants. The strongest sound in English is the vowel 'aw', the weakest is the consonant 'th'; hence the word 'thaw' contains the greatest possible intensity variation, about 30 dB. The level of intensity varies constantly as we make our voices louder or quieter, but the relative difference between the sounds remains the same, whatever intensity is used.

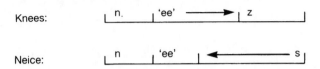

Fig. 4.9 Vowel length is influenced by the length of the following consonants. The vowel in 'knees' is much longer than the same sound in 'niece', where the following consonant is long.

The average intensity of speech ranges from about 35 dBA to 65 dBA, that is it has a range of about 30 dB. The following list gives the approximate order for intensity from loudest to quietest speech sounds:

1. vowels, such as 'aw', 'ee';
2. vowel-like, such as 'l', 'r';
3. nasals, such as 'm', 'n';
4. voiced plosives and fricatives, such as 'v', 'g';
5. voiceless plosives, such as 'p', 't';
6. voiceless fricatives, such as 'f', 's'.

This varying intensity can also be shown in the 'average speech spectrum', which is sometimes drawn on the audiogram, where the average range of speech energy, expressed in dBHL, can be used to predict what a hearing impaired individual is likely to hear. This is shown in Figure 8.4.

4.5 HEARING LOSS AND SPEECH PERCEPTION

Most hearing impaired people have hearing for vowels but unfortunately vowels give little meaning to the sentence. Although a gross over-simplification, it is often helpful to think of the written pattern, and if a sentence is presented without consonants it is very difficult to understand:

$$\_ \_ e \ \_ u \_ \ i \_ \ \_ \_ i \_ i \_ \_$$

If the same sentence is presented without vowels, the picture is much clearer:

$$Th \_ \ s \_ n \ \_ s \ sh \_ n \_ ng$$

The high information content of consonants is unfortunate as they are largely also high in frequency and low in intensity, making it difficult for the hearing impaired to perceive speech clearly. Hearing for vowels is not enough, but even if hearing is defective, speech can be a successful means of communication because it is so rich in redundant cues.

To some extent, it is possible to predict what a person can hear from the audiogram.

(a) Vowels

1. To hear vowels, the first two formants must be perceived and therefore hearing to 3 kHz is needed.
2. Hearing up to 2 kHz only, cuts off formant two and therefore creates difficulties in hearing front vowels 'ee' and 'i'.
3. With hearing only below 1 kHz, vowel discrimination becomes very difficult as nearly all of the second formant is gone, but some back vowels can be discriminated.
4. With hearing only below 500 Hz, there remains a thread of pitch variation, and detection of whether a sound is voiced.

(b) Fricatives

Fricatives will only be heard with some high frequency hearing present since they have little energy below 2 kHz and to hear them adequately hearing up to at least 6 kHz is required.

(c) Plosives

These short bursts of sound are difficult to hear but cues are available in the preceding silence, or stop, in the length and in the transitions to the vowel formants. Hearing up to about 800 Hz is required to hear front plosives, mid-plosives are higher in frequency, needing hearing up to about 2 kHz, and back plosives higher still, up to about 4 kHz.

4.6 HEARING LOSS AND SPEECH PRODUCTION

Where hearing is available it is used not only to hear others but, unconsciously, to monitor the speaker's own speech. This is known as **auditory feedback**. A speaker hears his or her own speech partly by air conduction, but also all voiced sounds are heard by bone conduction. This is the reason why people may not immediately recognize their own voice when it is played back from a tape recorder – they are not used to hearing it by air conduction only.

If there is a hearing impairment auditory feedback is less reliable, and individuals with a sensorineural loss usually speak loudly, so they can hear themselves. Those with a conductive loss often speak too quietly because they continue to hear their own voice well by bone conduction, while hearing other people more quietly by air conduction. With a severe hearing loss, monitoring speech through auditory feedback becomes very difficult and speech production may be severely affected. Some profoundly deaf people use their nasal and sinus cavities to resonate the lower frequency sounds, which may be audible to them. Other feedback mechanisms also become of greater importance. **Tactile feedback** uses the sense of touch and an unconscious knowledge of where the speech organs should be positioned. The motion of the muscles and the joints can also be monitored, and this is known as **kinaesthetic** or **proprioceptive feedback**.

4.7 SUMMARY

Speech perception is really the recognition of patterns. All languages have a high degree of redundancy, which makes them easy to understand. The speech message contains many redundant cues, both acoustic and non-acoustic, on which a person can draw when the need arises. The hearing impaired must process language in a different way, evolving their own set of cues to help them. It is possible to predict, to some extent, what a person can hear from their audiogram; it is much more difficult to predict how they will use what they may hear, because each person varies in their sensitivity to the cues available.

FURTHER READING

Moore, B.C.J. (1989) *An Introduction to the Psychology of Hearing*, 3rd edn, Academic Press, London, pp. 254–84.
Sanders, D. (1982) *Aural Rehabilitation*, Parts I and II, Prentice-Hall, Englewood Cliffs, New Jersey.
Schow, R.L. and Nerbonne, M.A. (1989) *Introduction to Aural Rehabilitation*, 2nd edn, Pro-Ed, Austen, Texas.

The hearing aid system

5

5.1 THE BASIC COMPONENTS OF A HEARING AID

5.1.1 INTRODUCTION

A hearing aid is simply a miniature public address system (Figure 5.1). Sound waves strike a microphone, which converts energy into a weak electrical signal. The signal is fed into an amplifier. The amplifier signal is used to drive a loudspeaker, which converts the electrical signal back into acoustic energy. The sound waves generated are then 'piped' into the external ear canal. The acoustic energy delivered to the ear is always greater than that received by the microphone. This additional energy is provided by the battery.

Hearing aids are signal processors in that they alter the input signal with the aim of improving it for the user. Unfortunately, it is not yet possible to increase the signal strength without introducing some distortion, that is the output signal differs from the input signal in parameters other than intensity. In some applications the signal is deliberately modified with the aim of improving speech intelligibility.

The following sections describe the basic components used in a simple hearing aid system.

5.1.2 THE MICROPHONE

(a) Introduction

A transducer is a device that converts energy from one form to another form. A microphone is a transducer. It converts acoustic energy into electrical power, either by direct contact with the vibrating source or, more usually, by intercepting sound waves radiating from a source.

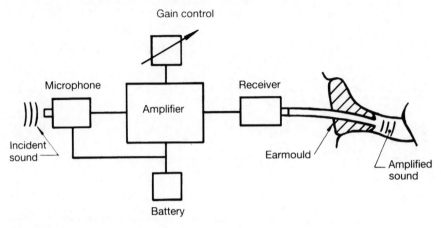

Fig. 5.1 A hearing aid system.

Microphones that pick up sound waves from the air have diaphragms to collect the acoustic energy. They fall into two basic categories according to whether one or both sides of the diaphragm are exposed to sound waves.

Pressure microphones

Pressure operated microphones have only one side of their diaphragm exposed to the sound waves. The other side is sealed off, except for a small aperture to allow the atmospheric pressure to equalize on both sides on a long-term basis (like the Eustachian tube in the ear). These microphones respond to minute variations in the surrounding air pressure. They therefore operate irrespective of the direction of the sound source, unless their physical characteristics dictate otherwise, and are said to be omnidirectional.

Pressure gradient microphones

Microphones that have both sides of their diaphragms exposed to the sound waves operate by virtue of the difference in pressure existing between the front and the back at any given moment. This difference is a function of the different path length for the sound waves between the front and the back of the diaphragm. Obviously this path length difference will vary with the angle of incidence; this type of microphone has therefore a directional response.

(b) Types of microphones

There are four main types of microphone.

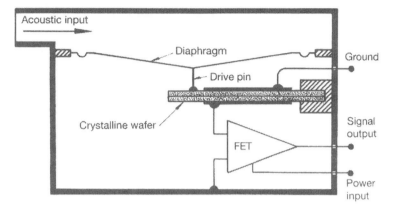

Fig. 5.2 A piezo-electric (crystal) microphone. (After Davis and Silverman, 1978).

The carbon microphone

In the carbon microphone sound pressure variations, acting on a diaphragm, are applied to a collection of carbon granules, thereby varying their resistance to an electrical current due to an applied voltage. This type of microphone has a high output and a non-linear characteristic, which tends to mute low level noise and saturate when subjected to very loud sounds. It is thus very suitable for use in telephones but, due to its high noise level and variable output, is not often used for other purposes.

The piezo-electric (crystal) microphone

The crystal microphone works on the principle that certain crystalline materials such as quartz generate small electrical signals when physically stressed. Various configurations are produced in which the movement of a diaphragm causes a wafer of the crystal to either twist or bend (Figure 5.2).

Crystal microphones have a very high impedance, and when connected to an amplifier (usually a field effect transistor – FET) with too low an input impedance will result in the loss of the high frequency response. Low frequency response is generally good, and the very nature of the design means that they are robust and stable.

The dynamic (moving coil) microphone

The dynamic or moving coil microphone consists of a fine coil of wire around a balanced armature, which is attached to a diaphragm and suspended in a permanent magnetic field (Figure 5.3). When sound

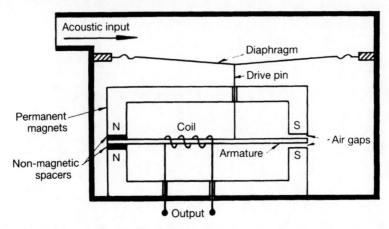

Fig. 5.3 A dynamic (moving coil/balanced armature) microphone. (After Davis and Silverman, 1978).

pressure waves hit the diaphragm, the diaphragm moves the coil in proportion to the wave intensity and causes the coil to cut across the fixed lines of magnetic flux supplied by the permanent magnet. The amplitude of the current flow induced in the coil is proportional to the distance moved and the speed of movement.

In order to reduce unwanted resonance (vibration) of the diaphragm, the coil must be kept light, consequently the impedance of moving coil microphones tends to be low. Stray magnetic fields can cause interference.

The capacitor (condenser) microphone

The capacitor microphone uses electrostatic principles rather than the electromagnetic principles used by a dynamic microphone. The microphone consists of two very thin plates, one moveable and one fixed, which form a capacitor (formerly called a condenser, hence the name condenser microphone).

Variations in the sound pressure cause the diaphragm to move with respect to the back plate so that the capacitance varies in relation to the sound wave. The capacitance is determined by the composition and the surface area of the plates (which are fixed), the dielectric or substance between the plates (which is air and fixed), and the distance between the plates (which varies with sound pressure).

In order to obtain an output, the variable capacitance must be turned into an electromotive force (emf). This is done by applying a polarizing potential through a high resistance. Variations in capacitance caused by the movement of the diaphragm are thus converted into a voltage

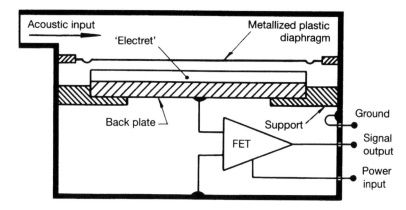

Fig. 5.4 An electret microphone. (After Davis and Silverman, 1978).

across the resistor which is then applied to an amplifier (usually an FET).

Some capacitor microphones employ electret diaphragms (Figure 5.4). These are commonly known as 'electret microphones'. The term electret describes a dielectric substance that exhibits a continuing polarization after an electric field is applied and then withdrawn. The electret polarization is analogous to the magnetic retention of a permanent magnet.

From the viewpoint of a designer, a significant advantage of the electret principle is that it obviates the need to supply the capacitor/diaphragm with a polarizing voltage. Compared to the conventional capacitor microphone the electret offers a potentially higher signal-to-noise ratio, is less susceptible to arcing, and exhibits excellent frequency response characteristics. However, the performance tends to deteriorate with time. The electret microphone is the one most commonly used in modern hearing aids. It is particularly suitable for miniaturization.

(c) Directional microphones

Microphones that have two sound entry ports (Figure 5.5), are known as directional. Sound from the front is given prominence over that from the rear, by the inclusion of a time delay network, so that sound from the rear is slightly delayed. If the delay is such that sound from the rear enters both sound ports at the same time, the sound waves will cancel each other out. In addition, some low frequency reduction is built into the microphone.

All hearing aids worn at the ear are directional to some extent, although a 'directional hearing aid' may be considered advantageous where a binaural hearing aid fitting is not possible. The degree of extra

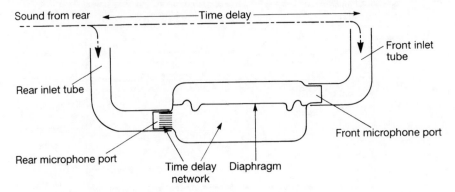

Fig. 5.5 A directional microphone.

benefit afforded by a directional microphone in comparison with an omnidirectional microphone, at the ear, is small and is probably only about 3 dB or 4 dB in reverberant conditions (Madison and Hawkins, 1983).

5.1.3 THE AMPLIFIER

(a) Introduction

Amplifiers are one of the most common of all electric building blocks. By definition an amplifier is any circuit that provides gain, that is, a device that delivers a high energy output in relation to a small energy input. Of course, amplifiers do not produce energy! The energy source for the output power is an external one which, in the case of hearing aids, is a battery. It is useful to consider the amplifier as a control device; a small signal input controls an energy source such that it responds proportionately and provides a more powerful output.

Hearing aids are complex pieces of equipment, and contain many electronic components. Among these components is the important semiconductor device called the transistor. This device is an amplifier in itself, but it needs to be connected to many other transistors, and other components, to provide the sophisticated level of control and amplification demanded of a modern hearing aid.

The bi-polar junction transistor is an 'active' device that can be used to control the flow of current through a load resistor by means of a small power signal applied to its control terminal. One of the most common applications of the transistor is as a voltage amplifier.

Modern amplifier circuitry often employs the use of a field effect transistor (FET, also known as a 'unipolar' transistor). The FET is a semiconductor device that depends for its operation on the control of a current by an electric field. The FET acts as a pre-amplifier because it is able to amplify small signals that are too weak for direct transmission to the amplifier.

(b) Amplifier classification and specification

In order to describe the requirements of an electronic amplifier for an application it is necessary to specify certain parameters and its class of operation. Amplifiers can be described according to:

- the electrical quantity they amplify;
- the frequency range over which they amplify;
- their relative input and output impedance;
- the class of operation.

The 'class of operation' is of particular interest and is therefore considered in detail.

Class A

Class A operation of a power amplifying transistor is illustrated in Figure 5.6. With this class of operation the transistor is provided with a forward bias so that a current flows without any signal present. The bias current drain is related to the maximum current the receiver will handle. The bias, or no signal, current exists even when there is no signal input and remains independent of signal input level and of volume control setting. Theoretically, an efficiency of 50% is possible. However, actual operating efficiencies can be less than 25%.

When signals are present, the current drain fluctuates within certain defined limits, but the average drain is still the same. Battery life is therefore fairly predictable. In the case of hearing aids, the fact that the power from the battery is being constantly dissipated, even where there is no input signal, is a major disadvantage.

Class B

A true class B amplifier is one in which the transistor is biased so that zero current flows when no signal is present. However, the device conducts on only one half cycle of the input signal and, because of the need for a small forward bias to produce current flow and initial non-linearity of the characteristic, severe distortion of the half cycles occurs.

In high power hearing aids, a modified version of the class B amplifier is used. This modified version is correctly known as a class AB amplifier (Duncan, 1988), but is more commonly referred to simply as class B. In a class AB amplifier (see Figure 5.6) the transistor is

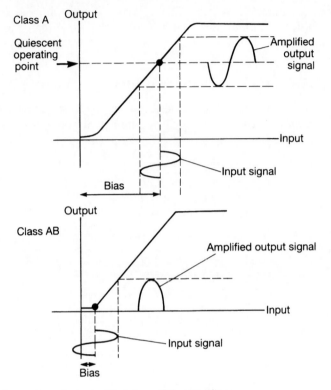

Fig. 5.6 Class A and class AB (class 'B') amplifiers.

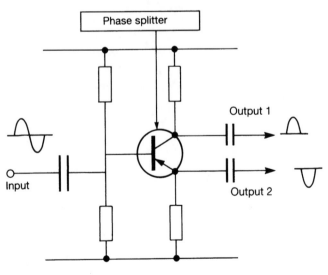

Fig. 5.7 A push–pull amplifier.

provided with a small amount of bias, just sufficient to allow the device to conduct slightly. Compared to a true class B, there is no distortion; however, there is a low current drain when no signal is present. When a signal passes through, the current drain depends on the required output level. The higher the output required, the higher will be the current drain.

To supply more power to the load than can be provided by a single-ended amplifier (single-ended means that only one output transistor is used), two transistors can be connected in a push–pull circuit. The output from the previous amplifier stages passes to a phase splitter, which separates the positive and negative phases of the signal. The positive phase is fed to one output transistor, the negative phase is fed to the second output transistor. The positive and negative phases are amplified separately and then combined to deliver a full wave to the receiver. A push–pull circuit is shown in Figure 5.7.

The advantages of class AB push–pull amplifiers are:

- a greater power output is possible for a given transistor;
- the efficiency is greater;
- there is negligible power loss when the input signal is zero;
- because of circuit symmetry, distortion is reduced since it may be shown that even harmonics cancel out.

The current drain is proportional to the output signal. As a result, the gain control setting directly affects battery life.

Class D

Class A, B and AB amplifiers increase the input signal without significantly altering its shape in the process. This is not so with the class D amplifier. The input signal is transformed into pulses, the time duration of which depends on the instantaneous amplitude of the signal.

The process begins with a triangular wave with a frequency that is at least ten times that of the input signal, typically 500 kHz. The input signal is then added to this triangular wave. The difference between the two signals emerges from a fast voltage comparator as a square wave with a duty cycle proportional to the amplitude. This square wave is then used to switch two output devices, which are either fully on or fully off, the difference being that the times they are on and the times they are off are varied so that the averaged effect can be made to replicate the input signal.

Class D amplifiers are very efficient, particularly at high gain, and can produce something like a 50% increase in battery life. Class D amplifiers are increasingly being used in more complex hearing aid circuits.

5.1.4 THE RECEIVER*

(a) Introduction

In principle, a receiver is a microphone in reverse. It converts the amplified signal into acoustic or sound energy, and transmits it to the ear. The receiver is the last, and often the weakest, link in the hearing aid system. Problems stem from the need to produce a relatively wide range of frequencies.

(b) Air conduction receivers

BTE and ITE receivers are generally of the balanced armature type (Figure 5.8). The alternating current output from the amplifier is fed to the coil surrounding the armature, which causes it to move within the permanent magnetic field. This movement is transferred to the diaphragm, which in turn generates sound pressure waves.

An external button receiver, as used with bodyworn aids, operates on a slightly different principle than that previously described. The signal current in a coil, which is fixed to a core of permeable magnetic metal, modulates the pull of a permanent magnet on a circular diaphragm made of thin magnetic metal. The modulation causes the diaphragm to vibrate, thus producing acoustic energy.

(c) Bone conduction receivers

Bone conduction receivers operate on the 'reaction' principle. A mass, free to vibrate inside an enclosed case, is caused to do so by a magnetic driving system (Figure 5.9). The vibrations are transmitted through the supporting spring to the case and then to the skin and the bony structure of the head. Essentially, a bone conduction receiver is the same as an external receiver, except that the diaphragm is fixed to the housing.

5.1.5 CUSTOMER CONTROLS

(a) Gain (volume) control

Most hearing aids have a dial or serrated wheel that serves as a gain control. It does not alter the input sound to the aid, but adjusts the

---

* In the hearing aid industry the output transducer is usually called the 'receiver', whereas in the audio industry it is usually called the 'loudspeaker'.

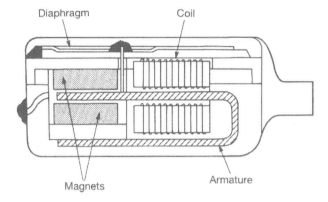

Fig. 5.8 A balanced armature air conduction receiver. (After Katz (1985).)

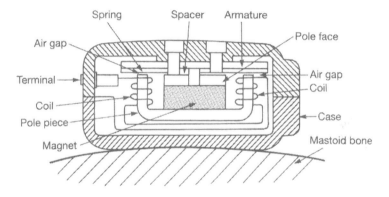

Fig. 5.9 A bone conduction receiver. (After Katz (1985).)

amount of amplification of the input signal. The gain control is a potentiometer, or variable resistor, consisting of a fixed circular carbon track. A sliding contact arm, connected to the dial, moves over the track and varies the resistance to input signal. An increase in resistance produces a decrease in amplification.

The relationship between the movement of the wheel and the increase in gain is **not** linear. Relatively little gain is available once the volume control is beyond 50% of its total range. Most of the gain (approximately 70%) is delivered in the lower half of the control, while only a limited amount is available in the top half. This is referred to as the 'taper effect'. Use of the upper half of the control may result in an unacceptably high increase in harmonic distortion.

(b) 'T' switch

A hearing aid can be equipped with a special circuit, which makes it sensitive to fluctuation in a given magnetic field. The circuit consists of a magnetic induction pickup coil mounted inside the case. A fluctuating magnetic field will generate a current in the coil, which is then used to produce acoustic energy. The coil takes the place of the microphone on the input component of the aid. If the 'T' position is chosen, the microphone is cut out of the circuit. For further information see section 11.3.2.

5.2 ELEMENTARY ELECTRICITY AND ELECTRONICS

5.2.1 THE ELEMENTARY PRINCIPLES OF ELECTRICAL CONDUCTION

All matter can be reduced to its atomic structure. An atom basically consists of a nucleus, which is positively charged, and orbiting electrons, which are negatively charged. The nucleus takes its positive charge from its protons. The number of protons is the same as the number of electrons, which gives a state of electrical balance.

It is a basic principle that opposite charges attract and like charges repel. In some materials the force of attraction is strong and the electrons cannot be detached from the nucleus. These materials are insulators. In other materials, the force of attraction is weak and the electrons are easily detached. These materials are conductors. Easily detached electrons are called free electrons. In order for free electrons to flow, an external force or electrical pressure must be applied. An electrical current is a flow of free electrons along a conductor.

If the current flows only in one direction, it is a direct current (DC), such as a current from a battery. If the source of electrical pressure constantly changes its polarity, from negative to positive, the current flow is alternating. Alternating current (AC) has a frequency; for example mains electricity changes its polarity 50 times per second, its frequency is therefore 50 Hz.

The direction and degree of AC current flow can be represented by a sine wave. This indicates a smooth flow of energy, first one way and then the other. This is the same representation as that used to show a pure-tone sound wave.

Current is measured in amperes (amps), although the small flow of current found in hearing aids is measured in thousandths of an amp – milliamperes. Electrical pressure is measured in volts. This is the force which drives the current around the circuit. Voltage is really a measure of how much energy is available to force the charge from one point to another. Voltage applied to a conductor in a circuit produces a current. If there were no other component in a circuit, the current flow would be controlled by the electrical pressure. Some resistance is essential to limit the current. Resistance can be likened to a tap that affects the mains water pressure and restricts the flow of water.

In a DC circuit, the type of impedance is called a resistor, which has the electrical property of resistance. A resistor, as its name suggests, resists or impedes the current flow. It acts as a constriction and allows the current to flow less easily. Resistance is measured directly in ohms, for which the Greek letter omega (Ω) is used as the symbol.

The controlled passage of current through a resistance is expressed in Ohm's Law, which states that the current (I) is directly proportional to the voltage (V).

The ratio of V to I for a particular conductor is called the resistance (R). This can be written as an equation:

$$R = \frac{V}{I}$$

For example:
(i) Calculate the resistance of a conductor if a voltage of 20 V produces a current of 4 amps.

$$R = \frac{V}{I} = \frac{20}{4} = 5\,\Omega$$

Resistance = 5 ohms

(ii) A potential of 12 V is applied to a resistor of 6 Ω. Calculate the current.

$$I = \frac{V}{R} = \frac{12}{6} = 2\,\text{amps}$$

The current = 2 amps

In the second example, the equation has been rearranged. A triangle arrangement is useful in remembering the possible variants (Figure 5.10).

A high resistance restricts the current to a low value; when resistance is small, the current is large. Resistance is one type of impedance found in DC circuits. Electrical impedance is the responsiveness, or lack of responsiveness, of an electrical circuit. In an AC circuit the type of impedance is called reactance. Capacitors are passive components used in hearing aids and have the property that the greater the impedance, the higher the frequency, as in a high-pass filter.

Transistors are active components, which work on the principle that a small current flowing into a base, controls a much larger current flowing into a collector.

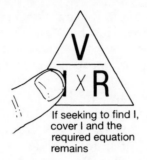

Fig. 5.10 A triangular aid to memory. (This triangle can be adapted for other formulae, such as those used to calculate battery life, or wavelength.)

5.3 SIGNAL PROCESSING

5.3.1 INTRODUCTION

Signal processing is a general term that includes everything beyond simple amplification (Wright, 1992). All hearing aids have some element of signal processing.

An electric current is more readily altered than an acoustic signal. Sound is therefore transduced to electrical energy before it is processed in some way. Many electronic options are available as user or dispenser modifications in addition to the main hearing aid components.

5.3.2. TONE CONTROLS

Tone control is a process that provides either high (Figure 5.11) or low frequency emphasis, and is similar to the treble (high frequency) and bass (low frequency) adjustments on a stereo system. The tone control is a filter network, usually between amplifier stages, which allows only the desired frequency to pass through the system. If high frequency emphasis is required, a high-pass filter (low frequencies filtered) is used, and conversely, for low frequency emphasis, a low-pass filter (high frequencies filtered) is employed. The terminology can be very confusing, for example:

- low-pass filter = low frequency emphasis = treble cut = high cut = L
- high-pass filter = high frequency emphasis = bass cut = low cut = H

Tone controls can be either a switch or a potentiometer (variable resistor), which is adjusted using a small screwdriver. In some cases the desired response can be specified and 'fixed' during manufacture,

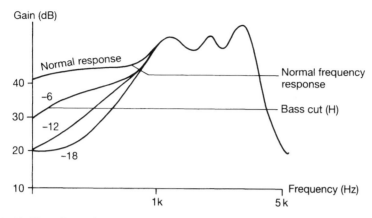

Fig. 5.11 The effect of a bass cut potentiometer on the frequency response. Reduction of the low frequencies provides a subjective high frequency emphasis.

or during programming in the case of computer programmable hearing aids.

5.3.3 VARIABLE OUTPUT LIMITING

All hearing aids have a maximum output above which they cannot reach whatever the input level or the volume control setting. This level depends upon the characteristics of the microphone and the receiver.

If the maximum output is such as to cause discomfort to the user, some form of output limiting should be used. There are two methods of limiting: peak clipping and automatic gain control.

(a) Peak clipping

Having been converted into electrical energy within the hearing aid, the intensity of a sound wave can be thought of as being represented by its amplitude (height). Peak clipping restricts the amplitude of the wave by cutting off its peaks and hence reducing its intensity (Figure 5.12). Whenever the peaks in the input signal exceed the pre-set maximum output limit, these peaks will be clipped off. Peak clipping distorts the waveform by producing something nearer to a square wave. This adds considerable harmonic and intermodulation distortion (section 7.3.5). The distortion produced by peak clipping has little effect on intelligibility because quiet sounds, including the information-carrying consonant sounds (section 4.5), remain unaltered; only intense sounds are reduced, but this may affect sound quality.

In a class A amplifier, only the peaks on one side are clipped, which

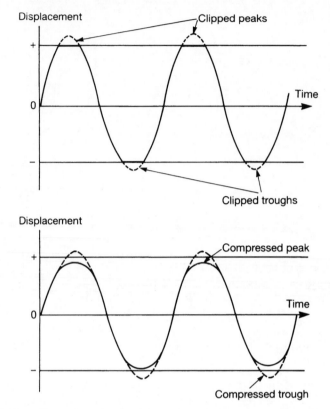

Fig. 5.12 The effect of peak clipping and compression on a waveform.

produces odd and even harmonics. In a class AB (or 'B') amplifier, clipping is symmetrical, producing only odd harmonics. The resulting sound quality is generally more acceptable, although peak clipping should not result in the aid constantly going into saturation. If this occurs the hearing aid audiologist should consider automatic gain control.

(b) Automatic gain control

Automatic gain control (AGC) is also called compression and automatic volume control (AVC). Automatic gain control limits the output of the aid by reducing its gain or volume in the presence of intense sounds.

The use of compression in a hearing aid is generally dependent on the user's dynamic range, that is the difference or span between his or her threshold of hearing and his or her uncomfortable loudness level. With severe recruitment, a narrow dynamic range will mean that if

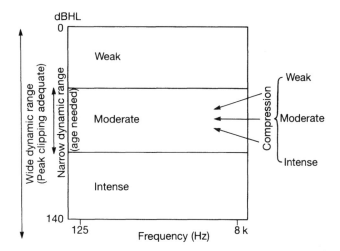

Fig. 5.13 Recruitment and the use of compression. In cases of recruitment, weak, moderate and intense signals all have to be compressed into a narrow dynamic range.

peak clipping alone is used to limit the output, weak sounds will not be heard, intense sounds will be too loud (Figure 5.13) and the aid will be in frequent saturation, causing distortion and loss of information from the signal. The function of compression is to control the gain automatically as the signal level changes. Up to a certain point, which is known as the kneepoint, the gain increases linearly, that is a 1 dB increase in input results in a 1 dB increase in output. Beyond this point, the gain is automatically reduced as the sound level increases, 'compressing' the signal and avoiding saturation (Figure 5.14). Thus beyond the compression threshold or kneepoint, a 1 dB increase in input may result in, for example, a 0.5 dB increase in output. This produces a compression ratio of 2:1, that is the ratio of input change to output change. Compression aids may be obtained with different compression ratios.

Unlike peak clipping, compression has a finite onset and offset time, known as the attack and release times. Attack time is the length of time required for the controlling action to come into effect. Recovery or release time is the time taken to return to normal. The attack time should be as short as possible to provide protection quickly at the onset of an intense sound. The hearing aid should have its maximum output set such that it will provide protection against sudden intense sounds.

The release time has to be slower than the attack time to prevent the aid from having an audible 'flutter' as the gain adjusts with the rapid changes that occur in a speech signal. An attack time of 5 milliseconds and a release time of 50 milliseconds could be typical for a hearing

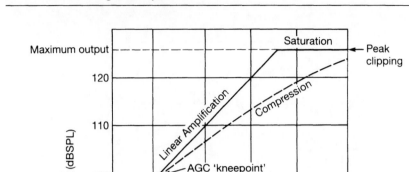

Fig. 5.14 An input–output graph for peak clipping and compression.

aid, although there are wide variations and adaptive compression is available with automatically varying release times.

Automatic gain control provides a feedback loop from a sampling point. Below the preset limit, or kneepoint, the feedback is too small to affect the circuit. When the kneepoint is reached the gain is automatically adjusted. Automatic gain control may act on response to the input sound level or the output sound level.

Output compression

Output compression acts to control the gain of the aid in such a way that the higher the signal intensity at the output stage of the amplifier, the lower will be the gain.

The kneepoint at which compression starts to operate depends upon the level of the output signal (Figure 5.15). Since the signal level is monitored after amplification, the maximum output is unaltered by the volume setting. Output compression is the simplest type of automatic gain control.

Input compression

Input compression differs in that the control threshold is part of the early stages of the amplifier. It is therefore the input signal level that acts to reduce the gain. The kneepoint is set on the input level, and

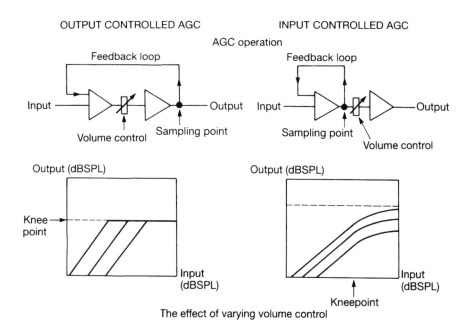

Fig. 5.15 The position and effect of the volume control in input and output AGC.

is independent of the volume control setting. Whatever the volume setting the kneepoint remains the same, but the maximum output will be reduced with lower volume settings (Figure 5.15). This is unlike output compression, where the maximum output is unchanged by the volume setting. Input compression results in better sound quality than output compression because it acts prior to amplification and therefore produces less distortion.

The choice between the various modes of output limiting depends upon the hearing loss and the client's acoustic environment (section 8.2.2(d)).

5.3.4 MULTICHANNEL SYSTEMS

A multichannel hearing aid facilitates the division of the frequency response into sections or bands, which can then be treated differently to provide a precise and complex frequency response curve that may be able to match the client's needs more closely. The need for a multichannel system may be indicated by an unusual audiogram shape, which would benefit from varying treatment in the different frequency regions, as for example a steeply falling graph with a region of good low frequency hearing.

The different channels may offer not only the facility to alter the gain, but also the output and any compression, in the various frequency bands. Where each channel has its own compression circuit, different attack and release times may be selected in the different bands. Shorter attack and release times are usually preferred in the higher frequencies than those used in the lower frequency bands. The kneepoint can also be altered in each frequency band to suit the user's dynamic range.

Twin channel aids may be relatively simple and their adjustment can be effected using trimmer potentiometers. More complex multichannel systems are often programmed using a small computer.

5.3.5 SIGNAL PROCESSING FOR NOISE REDUCTION

A hearing aid with a frequency response that is well-suited to a quiet environment may be quite inadequate in situations of noise. Many hearing aids therefore offer some switched in bass cut or 'noise suppression'. This means that the aid amplifies the full frequency response in quiet conditions, but operates a reduction in low frequency gain when it is necessary to reduce background noise. Some hearing aid systems provide automatic or adaptive signal processing (ASP) or automatic noise reduction (ANR), so that the aid automatically adapts to the level of background noise by reducing low frequency gain. When the background noise ceases, the aid returns to its normal state. This kind of ASP or ANR is only suited to clients who have a need for some low frequency gain; it cannot work where there is no gain in the low frequencies to reduce.

Certain ASP systems use the temporal as well as the frequency characteristics to differentiate background noise. Background noise tends to produce a fairly steady sound signal, unlike speech, which fluctuates rapidly. The aid may therefore reduce low frequency amplification in the presence of steady state input signals, or may reduce all steady state signals regardless of frequency.

Certain hearing aids offer a number of different frequency responses, which can be selected by the user according to the acoustic environment. The options may be selected using a switch, but a remote control is more usually employed where several options are available. Responses are most often programmed for quiet conditions, where the full frequency response is available, noisy conditions, where there will be some low frequency gain reduction, and for listening to music, where the low frequency gain is extended. A complex system does not suit every client; for some, the simpler systems are better. This is especially true when the client is unable to cope with the wider choice of options, or the extra rehabilitation that may be required.

5.4 SUMMARY

A hearing aid is comprised of four basic parts:

1. the microphone;
2. the amplifier;
3. the receiver, or the bone conduction transducer;
4. the power supply.

A transducer is a device to convert energy from one form to another form. In a hearing aid, the microphone and the receiver are the principle transducers.

There are four main types of microphones: carbon, piezo-electric, dynamic and capacitor microphones. Some capacitor microphones employ electret diaphragms. Electret is a term that describes a substance with a permanent electrical charge. Electret microphones are most widely used in hearing aids.

The diaphragm and the back plate of an electret microphone essentially form the two plates of a capacitor, separated by a small air space. The back plate is coated with an electret film, which has a permanent charge. Variation in sound pressure causes the diaphragm to move and thus varies the distance between the two plates. The varying distance causes a fluctuating voltage as an analogue of the acoustic signal. This is passed through a field effect transistor (FET) for pre-amplification, and then to the amplifier. The electret microphone has a wide, flat frequency response, is accurate and sensitive, has low internal noise and is easily miniaturized for use in hearing aids.

A receiver transduces electrical energy into acoustic energy (or mechanical vibration, in the case of a bone conduction aid), which is the reverse function of the microphone. Internal air conduction receivers are generally of the rocking or balanced armature type. External receivers, as for bodyworn aids, are more usually of the 'moving iron' type. Bone conduction receivers are essentially the same as the moving iron air conduction receiver, except that the metal diaphragm is directly connected to the receiver case, and therefore results in mechanical vibration.

Electronic modifications to the hearing aid that may be available include tone controls and output limiting. Multichannel systems divide up the frequency response into frequency bands, each of which is treated separately. Automatic or adaptive signal processing aids automatically adapt to the acoustic conditions in some way, most commonly by reducing the low frequency gain in conditions of background noise.

REFERENCES

Davis, H. and Silverman, S.R. (1978) *Hearing and Deafness*, Holt, Rinehart and Winston, New York.

Duncan, B. (1988) Which Amplifier Technology? *Studio Sound*, December Issue, 60–2.

Madison, T.K. and Hawkins, D.B. (1983) The Signal-to-Noise Ratio Advantage of Directional Microphones. *Hearing Instruments*, **34**(18), 49.

Wright, D. (1992) *Signal Processing Hearing Aids: A Preview*, Hearing Aid Audiology Group, British Society of Audiology, Reading.

FURTHER READING

Katz, J. (ed.) (1985) *Handbook of Clinical Audiology*, 3rd edn, Williams and Wilkins, Baltimore.

Lybarger, S. (1985) The Physical and Electroacoustic Characteristics of Hearing Aids. *Handbook of Clinical Audiology*, 3rd edn (ed J. Katz), Williams and Wilkins, Baltimore, pp. 849–83.

Tucker, I. and Nolan, M. (1984) *Educational Audiology*, Croom Helm, Beckenham.

PART TWO
The Practice Of Hearing Aid Audiology

The assessment procedure

6

6.1 PRE-SELECTION MANAGEMENT

6.1.1 CASE HISTORIES

The case history forms an important part of the early management of
the hearing impaired client. A structured interview establishes fundamental information, while at the same time allowing the hearing aid
audiologist to build up rapport, which begins to break down barriers
and reduce the client's fears.

Hearing impaired adults usually seek help only when they have
reached a stage at which they can no longer ignore their hearing loss.
The case history can provide an insight into the client's reasons for
attending, highlight particular areas of difficulty and reveal the client's
attitudes and expectations. Such information is generally most readily
obtained using an informal conversation approach, with careful listening, observation and gentle probing. A short form or list of questions
to act as a prompt (Figure 6.1) is often very helpful. The essential
information that should be recorded includes:

- the duration of the hearing loss;
- the rate of deterioration and any fluctuation in hearing levels;
- the cause of loss, if known, and any family history in relation to this;
- previous or current audiological, medical or surgical assessment or
  treatment;
- any conditions necessitating medical referral;
- previous or current experience with hearing aids;
- situations causing hearing and listening difficulty.

Any case history must attempt to identify those clients for whom
medical treatment or advice should be sought and the Hearing Aid

CASE HISTORY   CONFIDENTIAL

Date _____ Tel No _____ Age _____

Occupation _____ Previous Occupation _____

SYMPTOMS

Duration of hearing problem?_____ Cause?_____

Any deafness in family?_____

Any rapid worsening recently?_____ Did deafness occur suddenly?_____

Earache L/R _____ Discharge L/R _____ Tinnitus L/R _____ Headaches?_____

Vertigo?_____ Better ear L/R _____ Paracusis Willisi?_____

Exposure to loud noise?_____ Recruitment?_____

SURGICAL/MEDICAL RECORD

Seen Doctor?_____ ENT Specialist?_____ Name of Specialist _____

When?_____ Operation?_____ Type?_____ When?_____

Results_____

HEARING CORRECTION RECORD

Last hearing test?_____ by?_____ Using Aid?_____

Type?_____ How long?_____ Obtained from?_____

Results?_____

Why didn't you investigate your hearing problem before today?_____

AREA OF DIFFICULTY

Church   Theatre   Groups   Work   Meetings   Shopping

T.V.   Children   Car   Other_____

AURISCOPIC EXAMINATION

L ear_____ R ear_____

Continue over

Fig. 6.1 A typical case history form. (Courtesy of Ingrams Hearing Aids Ltd.)

Council (1990) provides guidance in clause six of its *Code of Practice*. This lists nine conditions that require referral for medical advice, and several of these can be discovered, or suspected, at the case history stage. The nine conditions are detailed below.

(a) Exposure to loud noise at work or elsewhere

Noise induced hearing loss (NIHL) may be caused by a single exposure to very high intensity noise (noise trauma) or by the effect of an otic blast injury, which is a combination of acoustic trauma and barotrauma. More usually, however, noise damage is caused by exposure to high levels of industrial noise over long periods of time. The effect of leisure noise, such as loud discothèques or personal cassette players, may add to the effect of noise at work.

Noise damage usually results in a temporary hearing loss, known as temporary threshold shift (TTS), which recovers to normal after a period away from the noise. After repeated exposure, however, the shift becomes permanent.

Referral for noise damage may lead to advice regarding ear protection, employer liability and compensation. Legislation (Health and Safety Executive, 1989) and increased public awareness mean that many clients will have already received advice prior to their visit to the hearing aid audiologist.

(b) Excessive wax in the ear

Cerumen, or wax, is a natural secretion that begins as light in colour, moist and sticky, but that dries out and darkens in time. Wax naturally works its way out of the ear unless abnormal conditions cause it to become hard and impacted. Previous problems may be revealed through the case history, but an otoscopic examination will be necessary to ascertain if the present level of wax is excessive. Referral is made to effect removal.

(c) Discharge from the ear

Discharge is a condition that may recur. The case history can be very important in identifying clients prone to discharging ears, for whom occluding the ears may induce or exacerbate discharge. Discharge may be caused by otitis externa or otitis media and, whenever discharge is present, extreme care must be taken to observe equipment sterilization and personal hygiene. Referral is necessary for relevant treatment.

(d) Vertigo

Vertigo is a hallucination of movement and refers to a vestibular balance disorder, not the unsteadiness of old age. Vertigo can be a symptom of several serious disorders, such as Menière's disorder or of a tumour affecting the VIII cranial nerve. Referral is therefore required for investigation.

(e) Earache

Earache, or otalgia, may be due to a wide variety of causes. The pain may be directly related to the ear or may be referred from some other part, such as from the neck or from the teeth. Medical referral is required for investigation and treatment.

(f) Deafness of short duration or sudden onset

Most deafness is gradually progressive in nature. Any loss of hearing that can correctly be termed as sudden should give rise to concern, as it may be symptomatic of a serious disorder.

Fluctuating hearing loss is a feature of many conductive problems, including Eustachian tube dysfunction; it may also be symptomatic of certain sensorineural conditions, such as Menière's disorder and vascular problems. Cases of sudden or fluctuating loss require referral for medical investigation, although the hearing aid audiologist should be aware that some cases may be non-organic in nature (section 12.4).

(g) Unilateral perceptive (sensorineural) deafness

A unilateral loss, or a marked difference between the loss in each ear, may be associated with specific causes such as a tumour. Medical attention is therefore urgently required unless the cause has already been ascertained, for example a unilateral loss due to mumps. (When undertaking audiometry, it will usually be necessary to mask the better ear to establish the true threshold of the poorer ear.)

(h) Conductive hearing loss

A conductive element to the hearing loss is indicated by an air–bone gap on the audiogram; there may also, of course, be an indication from the case history and from otoscopic examination. Most conductive losses are treatable, and a hearing aid system will therefore only be considered after medical advice has been sought.

(i) Tinnitus

Tinnitus is a complaint of noises in the head or ears, which frequently accompanies hearing loss, but which may occur on its own. If tinnitus is present, the client must be referred for further investigation. If medical treatment is not indicated, masking with hearing aids or tinnitus masking instruments may be effective (section 12.1).

The pre-audiometric assessment of the hearing impaired person is an important part of the auditory rehabilitation process. Discussion may help to break down any barriers to progress at later stages and help in establishing mutual understanding. Knowledge of the client's history may be particularly helpful if the client has received poor advice previously. A hearing aid audiologist, unless medically qualified, is not in a position to make a diagnosis or prescribe treatment, but the case history provides an opportunity to explore the client's hearing and communication difficulties, and may also reveal certain problems necessitating medical referral.

6.2 OTOSCOPY

6.2.1 INTRODUCTION

Otoscopy is usually performed prior to audiometry. Visual inspection of the ear is essential to detect abnormalities that should be referred to a medical practitioner, and to determine the size and shape of the pinna and external auditory meatus before taking impressions.

6.2.2 THE OTOSCOPE

An otoscope will provide both magnification and illumination. It should be supplied with at least three different-sized specula. The largest speculum that will fit comfortably into the external auditory meatus should be chosen from these, to provide a wide view of the eardrum, with as much illumination as possible.

The specula should be sterilized by an accepted method. Most hearing aid audiologists use a mixture of 20% sterilizing fluid with 80% water. The solution should be changed regularly, preferably daily. Specula should be cleaned thoroughly before being put in the solution and should be left there for at least half an hour before re-use. When required, they should be removed from the solution using tweezers and dried with tissues, ensuring that the tips of the specula are not handled.

When using the otoscope, it should be held in such a way as to minimize the possibility of discomfort or injury if the client moves. This can be achieved by holding the barrel of the otoscope like a pencil and resting a finger firmly but gently against the client's cheek or head. The barrel of the otoscope should not be held pointing downwards as it is more difficult to prevent the speculum accidentally being inserted deeper into the canal by a sudden movement of the head.

6.2.3 THE EXAMINATION

The client should be seated so as to be accessible. Ideally the hearing aid audiologist should also be seated to bring his or her eyeline to the level of the client's ear. All equipment required should be laid out in readiness on a clean towel, preferably white for reasons of hygiene.

The client should be given a simple explanation of the procedure. After washing his or her hands, the hearing aid audiologist should inspect the pinna and the surrounding area for abnormalities, such as signs of tenderness, skin disorder, deformity or previous surgery.

The external auditory meatus should be straightened by lifting the pinna upwards and backwards. If the client is a young child the angle of the meatus is likely to be more horizontal or downwards than that of the adult. In this case, therefore, the ear would be pulled gently downwards or horizontally backwards.

The correct speculum should be chosen by noting the size of the meatal entrance. Having connected the speculum to the otoscope, the speculum should be placed gently into the meatal entrance. The best view can be obtained by taking the eye down to be on a level with, or looking slightly upwards into, the lens, and moving not only the otoscope but also the eye as necessary. After inspection, the speculum should be cleaned and returned to the sterilizing solution.

Inspection with an otoscope should include viewing the external auditory meatus and the tympanic membrane. The meatus should be checked for signs of foreign bodies, wax, inflammation, growths and discharge. The tympanic membrane should be inspected for any variation from normal.

The normal tympanic membrane appears pale grey and semitransparent. On otoscopic examination the handle of the malleus can be seen extending downwards towards the centre of the drum. A cone of light extends from the umbo, following the direction of the jawline. This is light that is reflected back from the otoscope and is known as the 'light reflex'. The lateral process of the malleus can be seen as a white prominence at the upper end of the handle of the malleus, and the blood vessels which supply the tympanic membrane may also be seen. The tympanic membrane as viewed through an otoscope is outlined in Figure 6.2.

Inspection should include noting the colour of the tympanic mem-

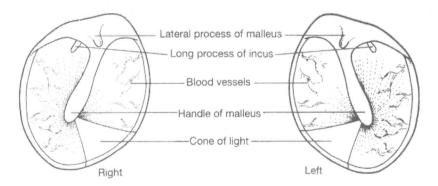

Lateral process of malleus

Long process of incus

Blood vessels

Handle of malleus

Cone of light

Right   Left

Fig. 6.2 The normal tympanic membrane as viewed through an otoscope.

brane, the presence and position of the light reflex, any scarring or perforations and any other abnormalities. Early signs of otitis media may be found at the otoscopic examination. If there is infection present the tympanic membrane will often appear very red. Failure of the Eustachian tube to aerate the middle ear adequately, whether due to infection or other cause, will result in retraction of the tympanic membrane, which will also appear dull. When fluid begins to collect in the middle ear, the tympanic membrane may begin to bulge outwards and the fluid may sometimes be seen. If the tympanic membrane perforates, the fluid will discharge into the external ear.

6.3 TUNING FORK TESTS

6.3.1 INTRODUCTION

Tuning forks may be used in simple brief tests to determine the type of hearing loss. The equipment is inexpensive, light, small and portable, and the results are reliable as far as the type of loss is concerned. The tests provide no reliable information with regard to the degree of hearing loss and the results are limited to the frequency of the tuning fork used. Tuning fork tests cannot be performed on patients whose loss is too severe to be able to hear the vibrations of the tines.

Tuning fork tests are widely used by otologists to provide early diagnostic information prior to audiometric assessment. They may be used when audiometry is not available, when a full audiometric test is not possible, or as a preliminary indicator of the condition.

A tuning fork is a simple device, made of steel, aluminium or magnesium, that vibrates when struck. Its prongs, or tines, move alternately away from and towards each other (Figure 1.1) and produce a relatively pure tone. The fork should not be struck heavily, or on a hard surface, since the tone would no longer be pure, as harmonics are introduced. Tuning forks for audiometric investigation require a flat base.

A tuning fork should be held by the stem and struck, about two-thirds of the way along the tines, on a rubber pad or on the knee or elbow. Alternatively, the fork may be plucked at the top of the tines.

The preferred frequency of fork to be used is 512 Hz (British Society of Audiology, 1987). Other frequencies may be used, but very high tones fade too quickly to be of much use, while very low tones may produce vibrotactile results, that is, they may be felt rather than heard. Whatever frequency is used, the results obtained apply only to that frequency.

Several tuning fork tests exist, but those most widely used are the

Weber and Rinne tests, which together provide a reliable indication of the type of hearing loss.

6.3.2 THE WEBER TEST

The Weber test is a test of lateralization; it establishes in which ear a tone is perceived.

The client is first asked if he has a poorer ear. The tuning fork is then struck, and its base placed on the midline, usually on the forehead, although it may be placed on the vertex, on the bridge of the nose, or on the teeth. A hand should be gently placed to support the back of the head.

The client is asked where he or she hears the tone.

1. With normal hearing or an equal loss the tone will be heard in the midline.
2. With a unilateral or an unequal sensorineural loss the tone will be heard in the better ear (Figure 6.3(A)).
3. With a unilateral or unequal conductive loss, the tone will be heard in the poorer ear! (Figure 6.3(B).) This is likely to occur because the better ear is able to hear background noise, which masks the tone to some extent. The ear with the conductive loss has no such interference and hears the tone clearly by bone conduction.

6.3.3 THE RINNE TEST

The Rinne test compares sensitivity by air conduction and bone conduction in one ear at a time.

The tuning fork is struck and held with the tines in line with, and about 25 mm from, the canal entrance for 2 seconds (Figure 6.4). The tuning fork is then held, without delay, so that the base is pressed

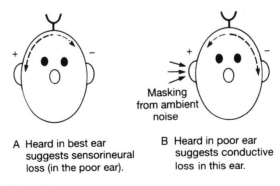

A Heard in best ear suggests sensorineural loss (in the poor ear).

B Heard in poor ear suggests conductive loss in this ear.

Fig. 6.3 The Weber Test.

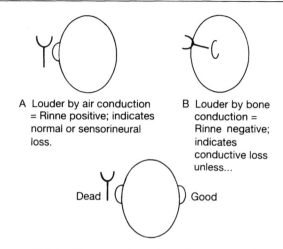

A Louder by air conduction
= Rinne positive; indicates
normal or sensorineural
loss.

B Louder by bone
conduction =
Rinne negative;
indicates
conductive loss
unless...

Dead   Good

...C False Rinne negative, where signal is cross-heard
by good cochlea on opposite side; suspected
when Weber test indicates sensorineural and
Rinne suggests conductive loss.

Fig. 6.4 The Rinne Test.

firmly against the mastoid, again for 2 seconds . A hand should be held against the opposite side of the head to provide counter-pressure.

The client is asked if he hears the tone louder at, or behind the ear.

1. With normal hearing, air conduction is more efficient than bone conduction; the tone is therefore heard loudest at the ear. The same result is obtained with most sensorineural losses. This is known as a Rinne positive.
2. With a conductive loss, the tone appears louder by bone conduction. This is a Rinne negative.
3. Where there is a 'dead' ear or a severe to profound sensorineural loss on the test side the tone may also appear louder by bone conduction. This is known as a false Rinne negative. This result is due to cross-hearing.

When a Rinne negative result appears to contradict the Weber test result, a false Rinne negative can be suspected.

Masking of the non-test ear may prevent cross-hearing but cannot be carried out accurately. Tragal rubbing is the most widely used method. A Barany box can be used but this produces high sound levels and should therefore only be used with care.

Tuning fork tests provide a quick indication of the type of hearing loss involved. They are not useful for determining the degree of hearing loss and should not be considered a substitute for pure-tone audiometry.

6.4 PRINCIPAL AUDIOMETRIC TESTS

6.4.1 PURE-TONE THRESHOLD DETERMINATION

The method described here is based on the British Society of Audiology's recommended procedure (British Society of Audiology, 1981) Test Method A. The threshold of hearing can be defined as the lowest level of a sound that is heard for 50% of the times it is presented.

(a) Signals

The test signals should be pure tones of 1 to 3 seconds duration with gaps of 1 to 3 seconds between signals. The tester should be careful to avoid a rhythmic presentation by using a wide variety of signal and gap lengths.

(b) Instructions

These should be as simple as possible to avoid confusing the client. In most cases, terms such as 'frequency' and 'pure-tone' should be avoided. All the client has to do is respond when a sound is heard, no matter how loud or quiet the sound is, and no matter in which ear it is heard. It must be stressed that it is important to respond to even the very quietest sounds when the client may not be absolutely sure that the sound was there. The importance of responding for the entire duration of the sound must also be stressed.

(c) Response

The client's response should be silent and not require excessive movement; a raised finger is acceptable but a raised hand is not. A response button and light arrangement is fitted on most audiometers, and this is ideal as pressing a button is a positive response from the client that requires minimal effort. The response should last as long as the signal. Although not ideal, in some cases a verbal response or a response in the form of a tap on the table may be necessary, for example, with young children, the very elderly, or those with mental handicaps.

(d) Threshold testing by air conduction

Any spectacles or large ear-rings should be removed so that the headphones fit firmly but without discomfort. The headphones should also be positioned carefully so that the test tones will be presented directly into the meatal entrance.

If the client reports a difference between ears, the better ear should be tested first. As it is usually an easily recognizable sound, 1 kHz should be tested first, followed by 2 kHz, 4 kHz, 8 kHz, 500 Hz and 250 Hz. The threshold at 1 kHz should be checked again for the first ear and if the apparent threshold is 5 dB different from the first value, the better value should be recorded. If the difference between the first value and the re-checked value is greater than 5 dB, then re-testing at other frequencies should be considered, the client first having been re-instructed. The intermediate or half-octave frequencies, that is, 750 Hz, 1.5 kHz, 3 kHz and 6 kHz, will normally not be tested unless there is a large difference (for example, 20 dB or more) between the results at two adjacent octave frequencies, or in cases of suspected noise damage where the audiogram may dip at 3 kHz or 6 kHz, or in all cases for medico-legal purposes.

The first tone presented should be well above threshold, without being uncomfortably loud, and this can be ascertained by asking the client if it was loud and clear. This lets the client know the type of sound being listened for, and the tester should ensure that the client responds correctly and for the full duration of this tone. With experience, the hearing aid audiologist will be able to predict an appropriate starting point. In most cases a 50 dBHL tone will be effective and this will rarely be too loud. However, if there is no response, or the client claims that the sound is rather quiet, then the signal should be raised by 20 dB and the test started again.

Each time the client hears a signal, the next signal should be presented at a level 10 dB lower, continuing until the level is below threshold and the client does not respond. After a null response the next signal should be 5 dB higher. This procedure must be strictly adhered to, down in 10 dB steps and up in 5 dB steps.

Threshold is defined as the lowest level, at that frequency, responded to at least half the time in the ascending mode, that is, following a 5 dB increase. At least two responses are required at the same level, in the ascending mode, to define threshold.

If the signals are presented in a rhythmic, and hence predictable, fashion clients may respond to signals actually below their threshold. Signals must be presented with no visual, auditory or other cues that might help clients guess when an 'inaudible' signal has been presented.

(e) Threshold testing by bone conduction

When testing by bone conduction, the bone conduction transducer is placed on the mastoid process behind the ear with the poorest air conduction threshold. The transducer must not touch the pinna. Only frequencies from 250 Hz to 4 kHz are used (section 6.5.2). While

250 Hz is included in the British Society of Audiology's recommended procedures (1981), this frequency is not always tested as responses may be due to feeling, rather than hearing, at low sound levels.

Thresholds for air conduction reflect the total hearing loss, whereas thresholds by bone conduction reflect the degree of sensorineural problem. The difference between the two, which is known as the air–bone gap, indicates the degree of any conductive element.

A purely conductive hearing loss produces thresholds by air conduction which are poorest in the low frequencies. The bone conduction thresholds should, theoretically, be 0 dBHL. However, this is not always true as the condition of the middle ear can have a slight effect on bone conduction sensitivity. For example, with otitis media, although low frequency hearing is good, there are often reduced high frequency thresholds, by bone conduction; with otosclerosis a dip in the bone conduction thresholds can often be seen at 2 kHz; this is known as Carhart's notch.

Signals routed by bone conduction will be conducted through the entire skull. It cannot therefore be said that the resultant thresholds necessarily apply to the ear behind which the bone conduction transducer is placed. If an unequal sensorineural loss exists bone conduction testing without masking will normally reflect the thresholds of the better cochlea.

Bone conduction with masking must be carried out whenever it is necessary to determine precisely the degree of sensorineural hearing loss in each ear separately.

The rules for masking are basically the same for bone conduction as for air conduction (section 6.4.2(b)). However, masking noise may be applied to the non-test ear either via a headphone or an insert receiver. An insert receiver has the advantage of being physically easier to use, and the masking levels required may be lower. Where headphones are used, it is very important to ensure that the test ear is not covered. Covering the test ear will appear to improve the bone conduction thresholds of that ear, due to the **occlusion effect**.

Occlusion occurs because a sound that is transmitted as a vibration

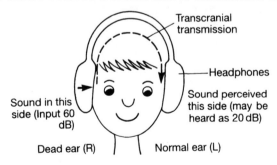

Fig. 6.5 The problem of cross-hearing.

through the skull not only travels to the cochlea directly, but will also reach the external auditory meatus by this route. Reflections from the walls of the canal enhance the sound, which is then passed via the tympanic membrane. Where there is a middle ear impairment, the occlusion effect may not be seen, as the transmission of sound through the middle ear is reduced.

6.4.2 MASKING

(a) Cross-hearing

Generally, a client's left and right ears can be tested separately by using headphones. However, in certain cases, there is a danger that the sound may cross the head, by bone conduction, to be perceived by a better ear on the opposite side to that being tested.

Air conducted sound has to be sufficiently intense to produce a bone conduction stimulus that will cross over. Some sound will be lost in crossing the head, so the signal will be heard at a quieter level on the opposite side. This is known as the transcranial transmission loss. The amount of sound lost in this way from an initially air conducted signal will be at least 40 dB, although on average it is more likely to be 60 dB and it can be even more.

Cross-hearing only causes a problem in audiometry when the ears have very different thresholds. In fact, it will not cause a problem unless the difference between the ears is at least 40 dB (the minimum transcranial transmission loss) (Figure 6.5).

It may help to clarify the situation to think of a client with one

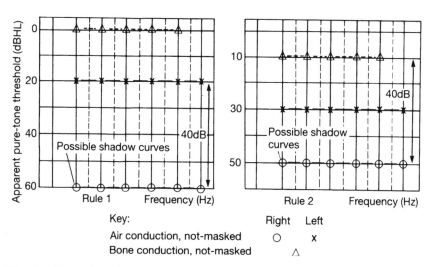

Fig. 6.6 Examples of audiograms showing possible shadow curves.

normal ear and one dead or profoundly deaf ear. A tone is fed into the dead ear and, since the client does not respond, the tone is raised. When the tone reaches a sufficient level, it will cross the skull, by bone conduction. The normal ear will now hear the tone as a very quiet sound and the client will respond. If the audiologist is not aware of the potential problem, he could think that it is the poorer ear which is responding.

On the audiogram, the threshold of the poorer ear often appears to follow the shape of the better threshold, hence it is called a shadow curve (Figure 6.6).

The problem of cross-hearing can be overcome by raising the threshold of the good ear so it can no longer respond, and the true threshold of the poorer ear can be determined. This is achieved by introducing a masking noise into the good ear.

(b) The rules for masking

Rule 1 – for air conduction tests

Where there is a difference of 40 dB or more between the air conduction thresholds of the two ears, at any frequency, then the air conduction test should be masked at that frequency. The better hearing ear receives the masking noise, and the worse ear is re-tested. The assumption is that the better hearing ear is hearing the air conduction test signal by cross-hearing via bone conduction. The transcranial transmission loss for air conduction signals is at least 40 dB. This can be thought of as the intensity required to set the skull into vibration.

Rule 2 – for bone conduction tests

Where the not-masked bone conduction threshold is more acute than the worst air conduction threshold by 10 dB or more, at any frequency, the bone conduction test for the worst ear must be masked at that frequency in order to obtain results for each ear separately.

It is possible that the not-masked bone conduction result refers to the ear with the worse air conduction threshold. If this is suspected then masked bone conduction thresholds will be required.

Cross-hearing is a major problem with bone conduction. The trans-cranial transmission loss with bone conduction is minimal, usually no more than 10 dB. This means that even if the difference between the two ears is as little as 10 dB, the bone conduction signal is likely to be heard more prominently in the better ear, wherever the vibrator is placed. Therefore it is necessary to mask on nearly all occasions where true bone conduction thresholds are required for an ear. Accurate, monaural bone conduction thresholds are often not required for suspected air–bone gaps as small as 10 dB, as specified in the above rule.

Rule 3 – for air conduction tests

Where rule 1 has not been applied, but where the not-masked bone conduction threshold is more acute by 40 dB or more than the not-masked air conduction threshold of the worst ear, the worst ear air conduction test will need to be masked.

The explanation for this rule is that cross-hearing is occurring by bone conduction. The air conduction headphone is sending sound directly to the contralateral inner ear through the head. Cross-hearing is occurring because the contralateral ear has acute inner ear hearing (that is, hearing by bone conduction) relative to the air conduction thresholds of the test ear. The transcranial transmission loss by this route is at least 40 dB.

(c) Method

The thresholds for the masking noise must be determined, so that the level of masking applied is appropriate. Too little masking will not be effective. If too much masking is applied cross-masking might occur, where the masking noise is heard in the test ear and interferes with the pure-tone threshold determination. Though it is important to be accurate, extreme precision in determining the threshold for masking is not required. It is not necessary to perform a test such as that used for finding the pure-tone threshold in order to establish a masking noise threshold. The threshold of masking is denoted M, in the British Society of Audiology's recommendations (1986). This is found by introducing the masking noise in steps, out of silence, and asking the client to indicate as soon as he can hear the 'rushing' noise. The audiologist can use any suitable wording of explanation.

For air conduction tests, masking will be applied via the contralateral headphone. For bone conduction tests, an insert masker should be used to present the masking noise, but if this is unavailable a headphone can be used. The earphone on the side of the test ear should be positioned on the side of the head and not over the ear, as this will result in false bone conduction thresholds due to occlusion. Care must also be taken to ensure that the headphones do not touch the bone conduction transducer.

Once the thresholds for masking have been established at the required frequencies, the client will need to be re-instructed to listen for, and respond to, the pure-tones while ignoring the masking noise, usually described as a rushing noise. Clients must not be told to expect the masking noise in one ear and the pure-tone in the other. If cross-hearing is occurring the client may be hearing the tone contralaterally, and it is often difficult for a client to identify the ear in which a sound was actually heard. Clients must simply respond to the tone, wherever and however faintly it is heard, and ignore the masking noise.

To start the masked threshold determination, masking noise is presented to the non-test ear at a level of 10 dB above the masking noise threshold, i.e. at M + 10 dB. In the presence of masking the pure-tone threshold is re-established. Some testers prefer to follow the usual and full pure-tone threshold method for this re-establishment, that is, presenting a tone at a level estimated to be well above threshold and reducing it in 10 dB steps until the threshold is found (section 6.4.1). Other testers simply present the tone at the previously determined, not-masked level to establish if it is still audible while the non-test ear is being masked; if not heard the tone level is increased until the threshold is found. The method used may depend on the client being tested.

Masking is then increased by 10 dB, to a level of M + 20 dB. The pure-tone threshold is again re-established by the chosen method. This procedure is repeated, with masking going up in 10 dB steps each time, until three pure-tone thresholds have been found at the same level for different levels of masking, and a masking level of at least M + 40 dB has been used.

A certain amount of error is permitted in the pure-tone threshold determination, and if three pure-tone thresholds differ from one another by no more than ±5 dB they are considered the same. This is the true, masked threshold.

In some cases it will not be possible to obtain a masked threshold where three results are the same for different levels of masking. In these cases the true threshold is said to be at or greater than the highest threshold determination for that frequency, and marked appropriately on the audiogram. Examples of cases where the masking test cannot be completed include:

- masking noise reaches an uncomfortably loud level;
- masking noise reaches the limit of the audiometer before the pure-tone threshold has been determined;
- the audiometer's pure-tone limit is reached before the threshold has been determined.

(d) A modified procedure for masking

1. Find the threshold for masking (M) in the non-test ear.
2. Increase the masking level by 20 dB (M + 20)

3. Present the test tone at its original intensity. (When testing by bone conduction, the original threshold must be re-checked at this point.)
4. If the test tone is heard, increase the masking by 10 dB.
5. Present the test tone again at the same intensity as step 3.
6. If the tone is still heard, increase the masking by a further 10 dB and present the tone again.
7. If the tone is heard, despite 20 dB increase in masking (M + 40), the original threshold is confirmed. Cross-hearing did not occur.
8. If increasing masking prevents hearing of the test tone, the tone must be increased.
9. The procedure is continued until two 10 dB increases in masking, that is three different levels, do not affect the audibility of the test tone.
10. In some cases it may not be possible to find the true threshold either because the client experiences discomfort, or because the limits of the audiometer are reached.
11. Masking at a level greater than 40 dB above the signal may itself cross over the head to the test ear. This is most likely to cause a problem where there is a conductive element of over 30 dB.

It is not usually necessary to mask at all frequencies. Two or three frequencies are usually quite sufficient; often, 1 kHz and either 2 kHz or 4 kHz are masked.

It is often helpful to record the results of masking while the procedure is being performed. This may be done using a masking diagram, or in simple columns (Table 6.1). In either case, the audiologist is looking for a 'plateau'. This is where three consecutive masking levels have no effect on the threshold (or no more than 5 dB). A simplified masking diagram, in which the plateau can be seen, is shown in Figure 6.7. If high levels of masking noise are necessary the noise should be turned down while the results are being recorded in order to avoid discomfort.

Table 6.1 An approach to recording masking results using columns

Frequency (kHz)	Pure-tone threshold (dB)	Masking (dB)
1	40	10
	not-masked	+20
		30
	50	30
	60	40
	70	50
	70 } Plateau	60
	70	70

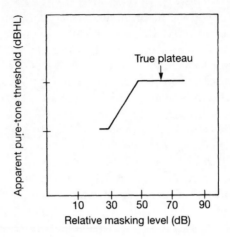

Fig. 6.7 Simplified masking diagram.

(e) Symbols

Where a true, masked air conduction threshold differs from the original not-masked value, and the not-masked value appears on the audiogram, the not-masked value is a shadow and the symbol should be shaded in. The true threshold should then be drawn on the audiogram.

If the masked and not-masked results are the same it is common in the UK to half-shade the symbol. Not-masked bone conduction results are identified by a triangle on the audiogram; masked bone conduction results use a special symbol:

O, X   True air conduction thresholds for right and left ears respectively, masked if appropriate.

●, X   Shadow, or possible shadow, results for right and left ears respectively. Suspect results, identified by the rules for masking, that are not checked by masking should always be identified as shadows.

◕, X   Masked air conduction thresholds that are the same as the not-masked thresholds. Could be left unshaded, but the half-shade indicates that masking has been performed.

△   Not-masked bone conduction thresholds.

[,]   True, masked bone conduction thresholds for right and left ears respectively.

A working audiogram may thus contain a plethora of results and symbols. Sometimes a final audiogram will be redrawn with the shadow results omitted, or the half-shaded air conduction symbols replaced with open symbols, so the chart shows simply those true results obtained with masking, and those for which masking was not required by the rules for masking.

(f) Types of masking noise

Masking is the raising of the threshold of hearing for one sound by the presence of another sound. In everyday life we are often aware of the effect of masking, for example, when trying to hear on the telephone against a background of noise from the television.

For the purposes of masking in pure-tone audiometry, wide band and narrow band noise are equally effective, but narrow band noise is preferred since it is less fatiguing. Narrow band noise should be centred on the frequency of the test tone (Figure 6.8) and have a band width of between one-third and one-half of an octave (British Society of Audiology, 1986). The reference levels for narrow band masking noise are specified in BS 7113 (British Standards Institution, 1989), amended in 1991.

Masking may also be required when carrying out speech audiometry. Speech-shaped or speech equivalent noise is normally used for this purpose. This type of noise is similar to pink noise in that it has its greatest intensity in the low frequencies.

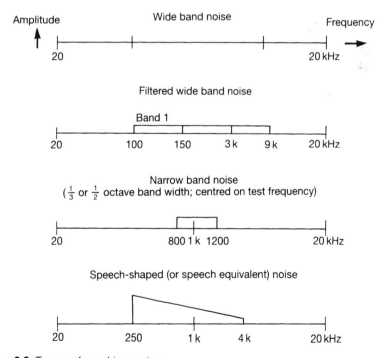

Fig. 6.8 Types of masking noise.

(g) Masking for bone conduction

A bone conducted signal is applied directly to the skull and can be picked up by either (or both) cochleae. The transcranial transmission loss by bone conduction is very small, between 0 dB and 15 dB approximately. Since there may be no transmission loss, cross-hearing must be assumed in every case.

If thresholds are required for each ear separately by bone conduction, masking will be needed on almost every occasion. This will provide accurate information about the type of loss in each ear. The only exception to the requirement for masking to ascertain this is where both of the air conduction thresholds and the not-masked bone conduction threshold are within 10 dB of each other. This represents a bilateral sensorineural loss of equal degree and masked bone conduction will provide no further information.

In practice, masked bone conduction is regularly required for diagnostic purposes. It is used less frequently for hearing aid selection, but ideally should be used (subject to the criteria discussed above) where a custom-built hearing aid is being prescribed.

6.4.3 DETERMINATION OF THE PURE-TONE UNCOMFORATBLE LOUDNESS LEVEL (ULL)

A client's dynamic range is bounded by the threshold of hearing and that level felt to be uncomfortable. A hearing aid system should fully utilize the dynamic range, and provide sufficient gain and output to make important sounds audible, up to but not exceeding the ULL. Accurate measurement of the ULL at different frequencies is consequently of great importance. The method described here is based on that of the British Society of Audiology (1987).

(a) Signals

The test signals will normally be pure-tones, but the method is equally applicable to warble tones and narrow band noise. Signals should be of approximately 1 second duration with gaps of approximately 1 second between signals.

(b) Instructions

The ULL is very subjective, and it is very important that the client understands what is required. A level felt to be simply 'unpleasant' will be lower than the ULL, but similarly the test is not intended to discover the threshold of pain; the concept of an 'uncomfortable' level must be stressed to the client; it is not a test of endurance.

(c) The test

The test should start at a level predicted to be comfortable, and the signals steadily increased in 5 dB steps until the client indicates that the ULL has been reached. The frequencies to be tested are 1 kHz, 2 kHz, 4 kHz and 500 Hz, in that order, testing one ear completely before starting on the other.

It may be necessary to repeat some frequencies after re-instructing the client, if the results are felt to be unreliable.

6.5 UNDERSTANDING AUDIOGRAMS

6.5.1 THE AUDIOGRAM

The results of pure-tone audiometric tests are plotted on a graph known as an audiogram. The audiogram form recommended by the British Society of Audiology (1989) is shown in Figure 6.9. This provides a separate graph for each ear, although in some cases the results from both left and right ears are plotted on one graph.

It is important to use standard symbols on an audiogram to avoid confusion. The standard symbol for the right ear is a circle, prefer-ably drawn in red, and for the left ear the symbol is a cross, preferably

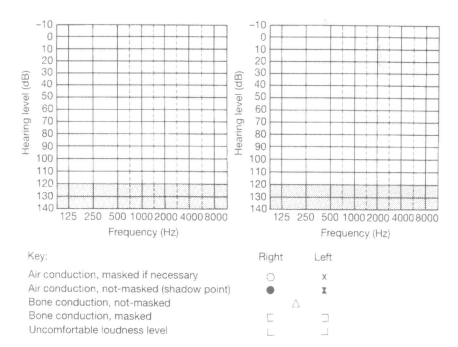

Fig. 6.9 The British Society of Audiology's recommended format for audio-grams. (After BSA (1989).)

drawn in green or blue. The symbols are joined up by a solid line of the appropriate colour. If the threshold shifts when masking is used, the symbol is completely shaded in. Where masking has been used but the threshold remains unchanged, the normal circle or cross is used. The fact that masking has been employed can be indicated, in writing, below the audiogram. Alternatively, the symbol can be half-shaded, which is a widely accepted variation from the recommended symbols.

Bone conduction (BC) thresholds are plotted with a triangular symbol, usually drawn in black. The BC results are drawn on the left or right graph according to the side on which the BC vibrator was placed. This indicates only the position of the vibrator, not which ear received the signal, since both ears will receive a bone conducted signal. Where masking has been used to obtain results from each ear separately, a square bracket is drawn, opening towards the test side. BC results are joined by a dotted line.

Uncomfortable loudness level is shown by an 'L' drawn to face towards the test side. When there is no response at the highest output for the frequency under test, an arrow, pointing downwards from the appropriate symbol, is drawn to indicate no response. The symbol is drawn at the maximum level tested.

6.5.2 AUDIOGRAM INTERPRETATION

A basic audiogram will show thresholds by air and bone conduction. The results should be interpreted in terms of:

- the total amount of hearing loss, that is, the loss by air conduction;
- the sensorineural element, that is, the loss by bone conduction;
- the conductive element, that is, the gap, if any, between the air conduction and bone conduction readings. This is known as the air–bone gap. Examples can be seen in Figure 6.10.

Sometimes in an audiometric test, the responses obtained may be due to feeling vibrations, rather than true hearing. This is a particular problem when testing by bone conduction, since the levels that may produce 'vibrotactile' results are much lower than by air conduction (Figure 6.11). At high frequencies, it is also possible for the tone to radiate from the bone conductor such that the client may hear by air conduction, again producing a false air–bone gap. Bone conduction is not tested beyond 4 kHz, but even at this frequency airborne signals may be heard near the maximum output of the audiometer. If the hearing aid audiologist is not aware of when there is a need to question the validity of test results, a sensorineural loss may be mistaken for a mixed loss.

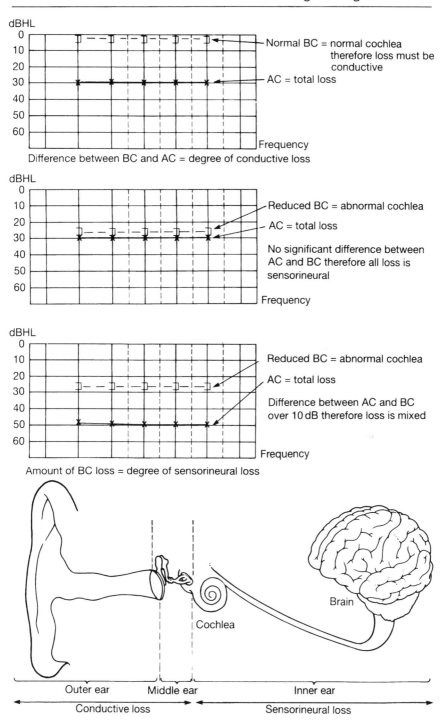

Fig. 6.10 Types and degrees of loss from the audiogram.

	Vibrotactile levels				
	250	500	1 k	2 k	4 k
BC	30 (5)	60 (35)	80 (65)	–	–
AC	95	115	125	130	–

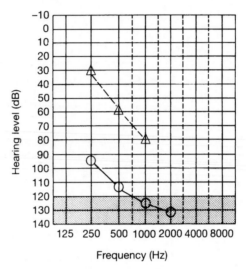

Fig. 6.11 Possible false audiometric results due to vibrotactile responses. Certain bone conduction transducers can elicit vibrotactile results at very low levels, indicated by the numbers given in brackets.

An audiogram that illustrates normal hearing will show a line of both air and bone conduction symbols along, or close to, the 0 dBHL line near the top of the audiogram. All three lines of the air and bone conduction symbols appearing within 10 dB of each other indicate a purely sensorineural loss in each ear (except in the case of normal hearing).

Where an air–bone gap is present, but air conduction readings in both ears are similar, it is usually unnecessary to obtain bone conduction readings for each ear separately for hearing aid fitting purposes. Where this information is required for diagnosis, or where the ears differ markedly from one another, bone conduction readings for each ear must be obtained by employing masking in the non-test ear. Masking for air conduction must be used if there is a gap of 40 dB or more between the not-masked bone conduction and the poorest air conduction readings on the audiogram.

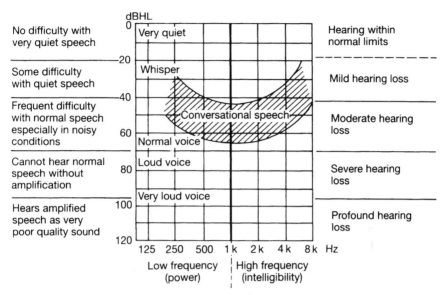

Fig. 6.12 Degree of hearing loss and its effect on hearing speech.

6.5.3 DESCRIPTION OF THE HEARING LOSS

It is often helpful to be able to describe the degree of hearing loss. There is no one standard description, but one classification recommended by the British Association of Teachers of the Deaf (Taylor and Bishop, 1991), which relates well to the effect on the hearing of speech is as follows (Figure 6.12):

• any hearing loss below 40 dBHL is described as mild loss;
• from 41 dBHL to 70 dBHL is described as a moderate loss;
• from 71 dBHL to 95 dBHL is described as a severe loss;
• greater than 95 dBHL is described as a profound loss.

The single figure of hearing loss can be obtained by taking an average over five frequencies, 250 Hz, 500 Hz, 1 kHz, 2 kHz and 4 kHz.

The concept of percentage is sometimes used to describe the degree of hearing loss. Percentage hearing loss is calculated according to formulae (King et al., 1992) for compensation claims, but the use of 'percentage' in place of dB to describe the loss to a client is incorrect. A 30 dB hearing loss, for example, is not a 30% impairment, neither is a 100 dB loss total hearing loss. A 100% impairment does not necessarily mean an ear has no useful residual hearing. The term 'percentage' hearing loss, for rehabilitation purposes, can be very misleading and should not be used.

A full description should include an indication of the audiometric configuration, which again is not standardized. The following terms are sometimes used:

- Flat, to indicate a loss that does not rise or fall more than 5 dB per octave.
- Gradually sloping, to indicate a loss that falls by 5 dB to 10 dB per octave.
- Precipitously or sharply falling, to indicate a loss that falls 15 dB or more per octave.
- Abruptly falling, to indicate a loss that is flat or gradual in the low frequency region, but then falls sharply. This configuration is also often referred to as a 'ski-slope', but this term is not recommended.
- Rising or reverse audiogram, to indicate a loss that increases by 5 dB or more per octave.
- Trough, to indicate a loss that falls in the midfrequency range (1 kHz–2 kHz) by 20 dB or more in comparison with the loss at 500 Hz and 4 kHz. Although not recommended, the American term 'cookie bite' is very descriptive for this shape of loss.

6.6 ROOM REQUIREMENTS FOR AUDIOMETRY

Background noise can have a significant effect on audiometric results, particularly those obtained by bone conduction. It is therefore necessary to reduce background noise to a level that will not elevate the hearing thresholds of the person under test. Ideally the room is specially constructed, but often audiometric tests are undertaken in less than ideal conditions, for example in the home situation. Background noise should be reduced as far as is practicable and the use of specially designed earphones or of insert receivers may further assist in its reduction. Where background noise is sufficiently high to have a possible effect on the thresholds, this information should be recorded on the audiogram. A sound-proof room is not a necessity for audiometry, but the noise level should be below that which would cause masking and threshold shift in someone with normal hearing.

Where a room is specially constructed for the purpose of audiometry, there are design recommendations that should be followed wherever possible (Department of Health and Social Security, 1974). The room should have an ambient noise level below 30 dBA. A prefabricated sound booth is sometimes used to guarantee a particular degree of sound attenuation. The booth must, however, be situated within a quiet room since it ensures only a certain degree of attenuation, not a particular sound level.

A booth that is to be used only for adults should be a minimum size of 1.2 m by 1 m with a height of 2 m, but preferably the room size should be at least 2.4 m by 2.4 m, with a height of 2 m. If children are to be tested, a room that is a minimum of 6.3 m by 4.8 m, with a height of 2 m is required. This allows space for free-field testing, and also for parents or other adults to be present.

A sound-treated room should be situated away from obvious sources of noise and should be isolated from the rest of the building. This can be achieved by building the room of brick with a concrete skin and cavity, thus using the effect of mass and of dead-air space. Vibrations from the building can be deadened by mounting the whole interior on rubber shock absorbers. Solid double doors should be used to exclude noise. Preferably, the doors should be lead-lined and should close with magnetic seals. Ventilation will be needed because the room will rapidly become hot and airless, but the noise from the ventilation system must be minimized using acoustic filters to act as baffles.

Tungsten lighting is preferable to fluorescent, which produces a hum, and if the latter is used the choke and starter should be mounted away from the room. If there are windows, double glazing should be used to reduce noise from outside. A much larger gap between the panes of glass is necessary than is required for heat retention. If the glass is 3 mm thick the gap should be at least 100 mm, and if the glass is 6 mm the gap should be at least 50 mm. In addition, where there is more than one window in the room, these should not be positioned opposite each other, as the creation of standing waves is more likely. This is important where free-field testing is carried out.

A room for audiometry must not only be quiet, but also have a low reverberation time, that is, there must be very little 'echo'. Rooms in which reverberation is exceptionally low are called anechoic chambers; these are very quiet and unnaturally 'dead', and are used only for research purposes. For audiometric purposes a reverberation time between 0.2 and 0.25 seconds is ideal. This should be achieved by covering the walls and floor with soft, sound-absorbent materials, such as acoustic tiles fixed on battens to the walls and ceiling and a thick foam-backed carpet on the floor. These will absorb sound and limit reverberation.

6.7 SUMMARY

Tuning fork tests provide a quick indication of type of loss. They should not be considered as a substitute for pure-tone audiometry. Pure-tone tests are used to provide accurate hearing threshold levels by air and bone conduction, together with determination of ULLs, which are important for hearing aid fitting.

Audiometric test results are recorded on a graph known as an audiogram. The audiologist must be able to interpret the results and to realize when false results may have been recorded, in particular those due to possible:

- cross-over of the signal;
- vibrotactile response;
- airborne radiation of a bone conducted signal.

Cross-hearing is a response from the non-test side, rather than from the ear under test. It will result in a shadow curve on the audiogram.

Masking is used whenever a shadow curve is suspected. It is also used to determine precisely the type of loss in each ear (using masked bone conduction).

A shadow reading should always be suspected if the gap between the two air conduction curves is 40 dB or more, or if the gap between the not-masked bone conduction and the poorer air conduction curve is 40 dB or more.

Background noise must be at a sufficiently low level not to worsen hearing thresholds. Low frequency noise can be excluded by solid construction; high frequency can be excluded by adequately sealing the room. Building-borne vibrations can be excluded by isolating the floor, suspending it on rubber shock absorbers. The ambient noise level achieved should be below 30 dBA.

Reverberation should be reduced through the use of sound absorbent materials, such as acoustic tiles. The reverberation time achieved should be between 0.2 and 0.25 seconds.

REFERENCES

British Society of Audiology (1981) Recommended Procedure for Pure-tone Audiometry using a Manually Operated Instrument. *British Journal of Audiology*, **15**, 213–16.

British Society of Audiology (1986) Recommendations for Masking in Pure-tone Threshold Audiometry. *British Journal of Audiology*, **20**, 307–14.

British Society of Audiology (1987) Recommended Procedure for Rinne and Weber Tuning Fork Tests. *British Journal of Audiology*, **21**, 229–30.

British Society of Audiology (1987) Recommended Procedure for Uncomfortable Loudness Level (ULL). *British Journal of Audiology*, **21**, 231.

British Society of Audiology (1989) Recommended Format for Audiogram Forms. *British Journal of Audiology*, **23**, 265–6.

British Standards Institution (1989) *BS 7113: Specification for Reference Levels for Narrow-band Masking Noise*. (Amended 1991.) British Standards Institution, London.

Department of Health and Social Security (1974) *Hospital ENT Services. A Design Guide*, Department of Health and Social Security.

Health and Safety Executive (1989) *Noise at Work*, HMSO, London.

Hearing Aid Council (1990) *The Hearing Aid Council Code of Practice, Examinations and Registration*, Hearing Aid Council, Milton Keynes.

King, P.F., Coles, R.R.A., Lutman, M.E. and Robinson, D.W. (1992) *Assessment of Hearing Disability: Guidelines for Medicolegal Practice*, Whurr Publishers, London.

Taylor, G. and Bishop, J. (1991) *Being Deaf: The Experience of Deafness*, Pinter, London.

FURTHER READING

Brooks, D.N. (1989) *Adult Aural Rehabilitation*, Chapman and Hall, London.

Hearing aids and their performance

7

7.1 INTRODUCTION

There are very few deaf people who have no hearing whatsoever; it is much more usual to have some remaining, or residual, hearing.

The residual hearing area can be illustrated on an audiogram as the area between the threshold of hearing and the point at which sound becomes uncomfortable. In effect, this is the useful hearing area. A hearing aid system is a device to enable a hearing impaired person to make maximum use of this residual hearing area and should provide:

- maximum speech clarity or intelligibility;
- maximum useful information from environmental sounds, such as the sound of the doorbell, or of an approaching car;
- minimum interference from unwanted background noise, particularly as hearing impairment restricts the ability to separate important sounds from background noise;
- minimum distortion; some distortion will occur when sound is amplified but this should be minimized so that it does not affect clarity or sound quality.

Several types of hearing aid system exist and selection from the range available involves weighing up the advantages and disadvantages of each type for the particular hearing impaired individual.

Air conduction hearing aids present amplified sound to the external ear and use the whole auditory system (Figure 7.1). Bone conduction hearing aids bypass the middle ear and are therefore useful in conditions that preclude the use of an air conduction system, for instance, if there is discharge from the ear, or the absence of an outer ear.

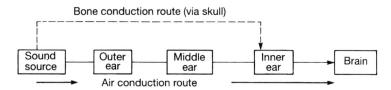

Fig. 7.1 The air conduction and bone conduction routes through the auditory system.

7.2 TYPES OF HEARING AID SYSTEM

7.2.1 AIR CONDUCTION SYSTEMS

(a) Bodyworn hearing aids

In a bodyworn hearing aid (Figure 7.2) the microphone, amplifier and batteries are all housed within the hearing aid case, which is linked by a cord to an external receiver. The receiver attaches to a solid earmould supplied with a ring and clip for this purpose.

Bodyworn hearing aids are relatively large and bulky and are usually

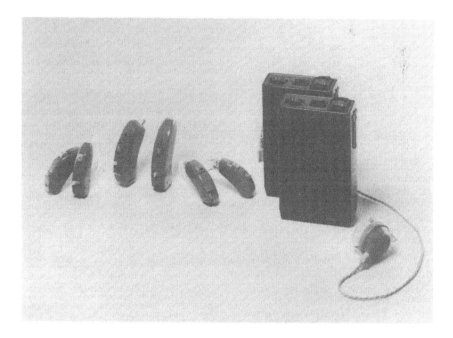

Fig. 7.2 A range of air conduction hearing aids. (Photograph courtesy of Viennatone UK/Bonochord Hearing Aids Ltd.)

worn monaurally, although a Y-cord can be used to deliver sound to both ears. This does not allow each ear to function independently and is not therefore a true binaural fitting. Binaural body aids are sometimes provided for children, although the unnatural position of the microphone, high up on the chest, minimizes differences in the sound signal arriving at each ear and therefore reduces the binaural advantage of improved direction and discrimination. Positioning on the chest will provide good reception of the user's voice. A bodyworn aid may also readily be held by another person who can then speak close to the microphone to improve sound reception.

The aid should not be placed under clothing as the clothes rubbing against the microphone would cause noise. If the aid is placed in the best position for sound reception, that is high up on the chest, spillage of food into the microphone can be a problem. This may be overcome by fitting a protective cover, which is known as a 'baby cover', but which is equally useful for elderly or physically disabled adults.

There are two groups for whom the use of bodyworn aids may be particularly advantageous:

1. For the very severely or profoundly deaf person, a bodyworn aid with its larger components can provide high gain and output, and a good low frequency response, which may be very important as an aid to lip-reading. The physical separation of the receiver from the microphone is a major factor in allowing the high gain to be utilized, as there is less risk of acoustic feedback. Acoustic feedback occurs when sound from the output leaks back to the microphone input, causing a high pitched whistle.
2. For those with manual dexterity problems – a group which includes not only the physically disabled but also the very young and the very old – the larger controls and accessible position of the bodyworn aid make adjustment easier, whether this is undertaken by the user or by a carer.

(b) Behind-the-ear hearing aids

Behind-the-ear (BTE) or postaural hearing aids are those in which all the components are housed in a case that is situated behind the pinna and linked to the meatus by a tube and earmould (Figure 7.2). BTE aids are available in a wide variety, both in terms of size and performance. They are usually fitted with forward-facing microphones, which allow full use to be made of the advantages of binaural hearing when two aids are worn. The position of the aid behind the ear may be uncomfortable for spectacle wearers and may not remain secure during active pursuits.

Various controls are available to facilitate modification of the hearing aid's performance and behind-the-ear aids provide an opportunity for early demonstration using temporary earfittings. All earfittings produce further changes in the response delivered to the ear, which may be desirable or undesirable. For instance, the external tubing adds undesirable peaks of resonance to the signal around 1 kHz and 2 kHz, while careful use of acoustic modifications such as vents and filters can greatly improve a hearing aid fitting. The effect of acoustic modifications is not precise but can be evaluated when the aid is worn.

(c) Spectacle hearing aids

Air conduction spectacle aids are those in which all the components are housed within the spectacle arm (Figure 7.3) and linked to the ear canal by a tube and earmould. They overcome problems of comfort and space behind the ear when wearing both hearing aids and spectacles. They are not widely used because in-the-ear aids provide another option, one which does not remove the hearing if the spectacles are taken off. Spectacle hearing aids can be supplied as complete systems or may be fitted to many of the spectacles, or spectacle fronts, obtained from an optician. Spectacle aids may also be used for contralateral

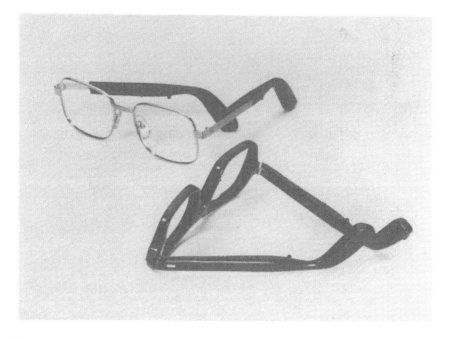

Fig. 7.3 Air conduction spectacle hearing aids. (Photograph courtesy of Viennatone UK/Bonochord Hearing Aids Ltd.)

routeing of signals (CROS). A basic CROS fitting may help in cases of unilateral hearing loss, where sound is carried from a very deaf ear for reception by the other, good ear.

(d) In-the-ear hearing aids

In-the-ear (ITE), also occasionally called intra-aural, hearing aids are those in which all the components are housed within the ear fitting itself, which is known as the shell of the aid. 'In-the-ear' is a generic term used to refer to the whole range of aids worn within the pinna but these are further differentiated into two main types (Figure 7.4):

1. Full shell in-the-ear hearing aids fill the entire concha of the ear. Variations can be obtained in which part of the full shell is cut away, such as half-shell and helix variations.
2. In-the-canal (ITC) hearing aids fit within the ear canal and may be situated near the canal entrance or well down the ear canal, near the eardrum, in which case they are known as deep canal or peri-tympanic hearing aids.

ITE and ITC hearing aids are available as simple insert aids used with a meatal tip but are most commonly provided with an individual shell

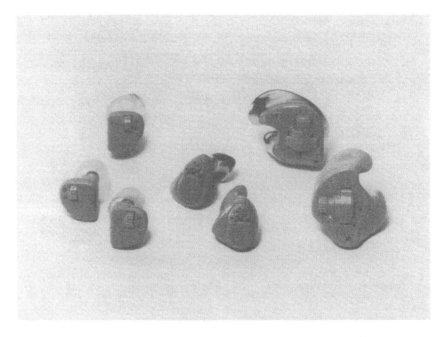

Fig. 7.4 A range of in-the-ear hearing aids. (Photograph courtesy of Viennatone UK/Bonochord Hearing Aids Ltd.)

made from an ear impression. The components can be standard or selected to produce an individual prescription hearing aid.

Most hearing aid users prefer an aid which is small and fits within the ear. ITC aids are the most inconspicuous but, whereas the manipulation of an ITE aid requires only a very simple movement (Upfold, May and Battaglia, 1990), the manipulation of the very small controls of an ITC aid is more difficult. The size of the aid also restricts the degree of modification which can be made by the hearing aid audiologist.

The amount of gain and output from the aid is restricted by its size, and the close proximity of microphone and receiver increases the likelihood of acoustic feedback. However, the position of an aid within the external ear makes it a very natural one, which allows it to take advantage of the natural forward focusing and acoustic properties of the ear. The further into the ear the microphone is positioned, the greater the natural benefit derived. Placement of the receiver within the ear canal also provides sound directly to the eardrum and the smaller the cavity between the sound outlet and the eardrum, the greater will be the sound intensity. These advantages of position will lead to an improvement in the amount of gain provided by the hearing aid of between 5 dB and 13 dB approximately, especially in the high frequency region (Sullivan, 1989), and since the ear fitting is an integral

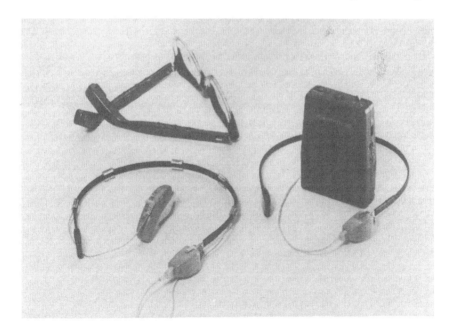

Fig. 7.5 A range of bone conduction hearing aids. (Photograph courtesy of Viennatone UK/Bonochord Hearing Aids Ltd.)

part of the hearing aid, the frequency response measured is that of the entire system.

7.2.2 BONE CONDUCTION HEARING AIDS

The major difference between air conduction and bone conduction hearing aids lies in the receiver. Whereas an air conduction aid has only to set air, a low impedance medium, into vibration, a bone conduction aid requires a great deal of energy to set the bone, a high impedance medium, into vibration. The bone conduction receiver is therefore large and rigid and fitted with firm pressure to the mastoid. Bone conduction hearing aids have poor high frequency response. They are used mainly for conductive hearing losses in which the ear must not or cannot be blocked by an earmould.

The mechanical transducer can be driven by a bodyworn or by a powerful postaural or spectacle hearing aid (Figure 7.5). They are generally not considered attractive and even the spectacle option must be provided with heavy frames, which may require frequent adjustment to maintain close contact with the mastoid.

7.3 SPECIFICATION AND PERFORMANCE

7.3.1 SPECIFICATION SHEETS

A specification is the detailed description of a hearing aid, which is normally presented as a specification or performance data sheet. This describes the hearing aid model in terms of its physical and electro-acoustic characteristics, together with any relevant information concerned with the method and conditions that result in the publication of that specification. The main function of the data sheet is to provide information in the form of tables and graphs illustrating the results of performance tests carried out to comply with the requirements of relevant standards. The standards aim to achieve a uniformity of hearing aid performance description that facilitates vaild comparison between different models. Small deviations from the specification are to be found in individual examples of any particular hearing aid model, and the degree of deviation acceptable is known as the tolerance.

When a purchaser receives a hearing aid from a manufacturer, the hearing aid's performance may be checked against that detailed on the specification, or on the individual data sheet that is delivered with a custom-made in-the-ear hearing aid (Figure 7.6). This is known as quality inspection on delivery and each hearing aid should perform within the tolerance stated by the manufacturer. Tolerances are not specified in the relevant British Standard.

STARKEY
Custom Data Sheet

This CRR/FRC CHS Hearing Aid
7193390565
was custom designed for the right ear of

MR.M. BRODERICK

ACTIVE HEARING,
THE HOLLIES,
88 HIGH STREET,
BOSTON SPA,
NR WETHERBY.

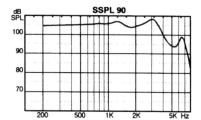

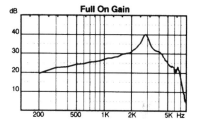

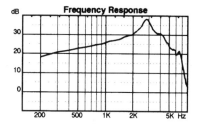

Matrix	107/35/10
Peak SSPL 90	108.3 dBSPL
H.F.A. SSPL 90	105.6 dBSPL
Peak Gain	40.0 dB
H.F.A. Gain 50	31.2 dB
Ref. Test Gain	29.9 dB
Eq. Input Noise	32.8 dBSPL
Frequency Range	200– 7300 Hz

Distortion: 100 Hz Filtering

500 Hz (70 dBSPL In)	3.8 %
800 Hz (70 dBSPL In)	3.6 %
1600 Hz (65 dBSPL In)	1.8 %

Battery Simulator:

Voltage	1.25 Volts
Impedance	2.5 Ω
Current	0.57 mA

10/01/93 08:45

QUALITY CONTROL
SIMPLY THE BEST.........K.W.
Est. battery life in 16 hour days with a 312 Zinc Air; 9 – 12 days.
All testing was performed in compliance with ANSI S3.22–1987

CRR Canal Resonance Response
CRR is characterized by a primary frequency
peak between 2.5 and 3 kHz. Placing the peak
in this region helps to restore the ear canal
resonance which is lost or diminished when a
hearing aid is inserted into the ear.

Fig. 7.6 An individual specification sheet for an ITE aid. (Courtesy of Starkey Ltd.)

The standards (British Standards Institution, 1988) provide for a number of different characteristics to be measured, including gain, maximum output, frequency response, harmonic distortion and internal noise. Measurements are intended to be used for the purpose of:

- technical comparison;
- evaluation;
- production control;

- delivery tolerances;
- selection for procurement;
- selection for pre-fitting;
- training and teaching.

7.3.2 GAIN

The acoustic gain of an aid is the amount of amplification it provides. In simple terms, it is the difference between the input and the output SPL. For example, if:

$$\begin{aligned}
\text{Input} \ &= 60\,\text{dBSPL} \\
\text{Output} &= 80\,\text{dBSPL} \\
\text{Gain} \ \ &= 20\,\text{dB}
\end{aligned}$$

Gain is always presented in dB without a suffix. It is measured under specified operating conditions and at a specified frequency or frequencies. The British Standard defines acoustic gain as:

> The difference between the sound pressure level developed in the acoustic coupler by the hearing aid and the sound pressure level measured at the test point.
>
> *British Standards Institution, 1984*

Gain is most usually presented as a single figure for 1 kHz or 1.6 kHz, or as an average of several frequencies. Alternatively, a frequency response curve showing how the gain varies across the frequency range is more informative.

A number of different types of acoustic gain are usually presented on a specification sheet. These include:

- Full-on gain – this is the gain with the volume control turned fully on.
- Maximum gain – this is the highest possible gain from the hearing aid. It is measured under specified conditions with an input that will not drive the aid into saturation, usually 60 dBSPL, and with the volume control fully on.
- Reference test gain represents more of a 'user volume'. This is measured with an input of 60 dBSPL, with the volume control set so that the output is 15 dB less than the maximum output (OSPL 90) at the reference test frequency. If the aid will not permit this, the full-on gain position should be used. The reference test frequency is normally 1.6 kHz, but where high tone hearing aids are in use 2.5 kHz may be more appropriate. This will be stated on the specification.

7.3.3 MAXIMUM OUTPUT

All hearing aids have a maximum output limit, which is the most the hearing aid can handle, due mainly to limitations imposed by the output stage of the hearing aid (the receiver). The maximum output may be referred to in a number of different ways, all of which have very similar meanings. These include:

- saturation sound pressure level (SSPL);
- saturation sound pressure level with an input of 90 dBSPL (SSPL 90);
- output sound pressure level (OSPL);
- output sound pressure level with an input of 90 dBSPL (OSPL 90);
- maximum power output (MPO);
- maximum output.

The British Standards define OSPL 90 as:

> The sound pressure level produced in an ear simulator with an input of 90 dB at the specified frequency (or frequencies), the gain control being in the full-on position and all other controls being set for maximum gain.

> *British Standards Institution, 1984*

Saturation is the condition in a circuit when an increase in the input signal produces no further increase in the output signal (Figure 7.7). Saturation sound pressure level is the highest possible SPL obtainable from the hearing aid. In order to measure this in the test situation, all the controls, including the volume, must be turned up to maximum and an acoustic signal must be produced that is sufficiently intense to drive the aid into saturation. This input signal is always 90 dBSPL.

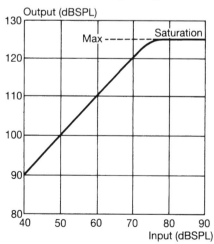

Fig. 7.7 An input–output graph demonstrating saturation of a hearing aid.

Saturation is the highest possible sound pressure level that an aid is capable of producing, and it can be specified at one or more frequencies.

7.3.4 FREQUENCY RESPONSE

The frequency response of a hearing aid is presented as a line on a graph that shows how the aid performs over the frequency range. It is defined in BS 6083: Part 0 (1984) as:

> The sound pressure level developed in an ear simulator by the hearing aid expressed as a function of frequency under specified conditions.

A frequency response may be obtained to show how the gain, or the output, varies with frequency and the term 'basic frequency response' may also be seen on a specification sheet. This illustrates the frequency response curve obtained at the reference test gain setting, with an input signal of 60 dBSPL.

7.3.5 AMPLITUDE NON-LINEARITY OR DISTORTION

An ideal hearing aid would produce an output that was identical to the input signal, only amplified. However, a hearing aid is not capable of doing this and when the output does not reproduce exactly the input, it is said to be distorted.

(a) Harmonic distortion

For the purpose of quality inspection of hearing aid performance on delivery only harmonic distortion is considered, since this is the easiest type of distortion to measure. It results when harmonics are present at the output that were not part of the input signal. Harmonics are multiples of the original frequency; for example, a pure tone of 2 kHz would add harmonics at 4 kHz, 6 kHz, 8 kHz and so on. The original tone, or fundamental frequency, is always the lowest frequency (Figure 7.8). It is also the first harmonic since harmonics are multiples. In the example given above:

$$\begin{aligned}
\text{The fundamental frequency} &= 2\,\text{kHz} \\
\text{The first harmonic} = 1 \times 2\,\text{kHz} &= 2\,\text{kHz} \\
\text{The second harmonic} = 2 \times 2\,\text{kHz} &= 4\,\text{kHz} \\
\text{The third harmonic} = 3 \times 2\,\text{kHz} &= 6\,\text{kHz}
\end{aligned}$$

The harmonic content decreases with increasing frequency and measurements usually only consider the second and third harmonics. These may be considered separately, or together as 'total harmonic distortion'.

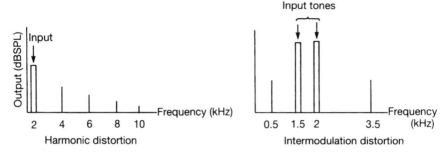

Fig. 7.8 Harmonic and intermodulation distortion.

A hearing aid should produce as little distortion as possible and this is expressed in one of two ways, as:

1. a distortion ratio, where the distortion product is given as the number of dB below the total output signal;
2. a distortion factor, where the distortion product is expressed as a percentage of the total output signal.

If the response curve rises 12 dB or more between any test frequency and its second harmonic, the measurement may be omitted.

There is no absolute agreed figure for maximum distortion but, as a general rule, a distortion ratio of 20 dB, or a distortion factor of 10%, is considered to be the maximum acceptable. Harmonic distortion increases as the hearing aid nears saturation point and it is therefore normally measured below this point, at the reference test position, or, in the clinic, it may be measured at the wearer's volume setting. Other forms of distortion, such as intermodulation distortion and transient distortion, are less frequently measured but may also affect the sound quality.

(b) Intermodulation distortion

This occurs (Figure 7.8) when there are two or more input signals and this results in additional frequencies, which are the arithmetic sum or difference of the input frequencies. Intermodulation products, unlike harmonics, occur not only above the frequency of the fundamental but also below. *BS 6083: Part 0* (1984) provides for the measurement of intermodulation distortion by the manufacturers; it is not a test undertaken for quality control on delivery.

(c) Transient distortion

Transient distortion, sometimes known as 'ringing', occurs when there is a rapid change in the signal such that the hearing aid cannot reproduce the sharp rise and fall times. A lingering of the sound often results, which may interfere with speech intelligibility, but the effect of this on the listener is not fully understood and there are no standards for measuring transient distortion.

7.3.6 EQUIVALENT INPUT NOISE LEVEL

Hearing aid electronics generate internal random noise, which poses a potential source of masking and must therefore be minimized. Internal noise may be analysed in one-third octave bands or it may be expressed as an equivalent input noise level. It is calculated with the aid set approximately to the reference test gain position.

To express the internal noise as an equivalent input noise level, the output sound pressure level with an input of 60 dBSPL is first noted. The output minus the input provides a measure of gain. The sound source of input is switched off. The sound pressure measured at this point is caused by internal noise. The equivalent input noise is calculated by subtracting the gain from the sound pressure caused by internal noise.

For example:

1. $OSPL_{60} = L_s = 100$ Input $60 = L_1$
2. $OSPL_0 = L_2 = 70$
3. Internal noise $-$ Gain $=$ Equivalent input noise level (L_N)

$L_N = L_2 - (L_S - L_1)$ where L_N = equivalent input noise level
$L_N = 70 - (100 - 60)$ L_2 = SPL caused by internal noise
$L_N = 70 - 40$ L_s = OSPL with input 60 dBSPL
$L_N = 30$ L_1 = input of 60 dBSPL

The internal noise generated in the example is equivalent to an input signal to the aid of 30 dBSPL. This measure applies only to essentially linear input/output conditions and where automatic gain control aids are involved, the input SPL may be reduced to ensure such conditions apply.

7.3.7 DYNAMIC OUTPUT CHARACTERISTICS OF AGC CIRCUITS

Automatic gain control (AGC) is employed to compress, or reduce, the dynamic range of the sound at the output. This prevents excessive output sound from the hearing aid from reaching the user's ear, while tending to preserve the waveform of the input signal. The dynamic characteristics of an AGC circuit, especially the attack and recovery times (see below), are important, and methods for the measurement of these and other electro-acoustical characteristics are given in BS 6083: Part 2 (1984) (Figure 7.9).

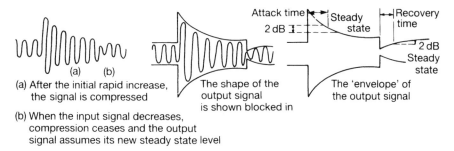

(a) After the initial rapid increase, the signal is compressed

(b) When the input signal decreases, compression ceases and the output signal assumes its new steady state level

The shape of the output signal is shown blocked in

The 'envelope' of the output signal

Fig. 7.9 The effect of compression on the output signal. (After BS 6083: Part 2 (1984).)

Automatic gain control is not instantaneous and the **attack time** is the time interval it takes for the AGC circuit to stabilize when there is a sudden increase in input signal. The stabilized level is known as the steady state.

Conversely, the **recovery time** is the time interval it takes for the AGC circuits to stabilize when the input signal is abruptly reduced. Both the attack and the recovery times are recorded as the time taken, when the signal is altered by a stated number of decibels, for the output to reach within 2 dB of its steady state level.

Attack times should be as short as possible to avoid sudden loud sounds from being amplified to the extent that uncomfortable hearing occurs. An attack time of less than 10 milliseconds is ideal since the human ear cannot perceive temporal changes of less than 10 milliseconds (Pollack, 1988).

Short recovery times, however, may cause considerable distortion and the listener may hear an audible 'flutter' as the compression circuit reacts to the variations in intensity that occur in speech at normal levels. Release times are normally greater than 30 milliseconds in order to avoid 'flutter' but shorter than 150 milliseconds to maintain speech intelligibility.

7.4 HEARING AID STANDARDS

In the early days of electronic hearing aids manufacturers set their own standards and it was impossible to compare different models by looking at the data provided. As the number of hearing aids available grew, it became increasingly important that hearing aid measurements be standardized, and in 1959 the International Electrotechnical Commission (IEC) produced the first European standards. Unfortunately, standards can still be confusing because there are major differences between European and American standards. Standards are constantly revised and updated. In practice this means that the date, as well as the number, of the standard used on a specification sheet should be noted. The main standards are:

1. European
   IEC   International Electrotechnical Commission.
   BSI   British Standards Institution. British Standards are generally IEC standards adopted and renumbered but retaining their original content. BS 6083 is an important standard relating to hearing aids; it is identical to IEC 118 and consists of a number of parts which are listed at the end of this chapter, in further reading.
2. American
   HAIC   Hearing Aid Industry Conference (1961). These early standards have mostly been superseded by ANSI, but are still in limited use.
   ANSI   American National Standards Institute.

HAIC specifications relate to average values over three test frequencies: 500 Hz, 1 kHz and 2 kHz.

- HAIC gain is an average value derived from the maximum gain at each of the three test frequencies.

Table 7.1 An outline comparison of certain hearing aid tests drawn from British and American standards (Source: ANSI 5322 (1987))

Characteristic	Input (dBSPL)	Frequency (Hz)	Volume control	Basic ANSI differences
OSPL90	90	200–8 k	Full-on	Entitled SSPL90; frequency range if used 200–5 kHz; tend to give as an average of 1 k, 1.6 k and 2.5 kHz
Full-on acoustic gain	Usually 60	200–8 k	Full-on	Tend to give as an average of 1 k, 1.6 k and 2.5 kHz
Reference test gain	60	Usually 1.6 k	15 dB less than OSPL90	17 dB less than average SSPL90
Frequency response curve	Usually 60	200–8 k	Reference test position	200–5 kHz
Total harmonic distortion	70	200–5 k	Reference test position	Measured at 500, 800 and 1.6 kHz presented as percentage

- HAIC output is an average value derived from the maximum output at each of the three test frequencies.
- HAIC frequency range provides for a standard method of defining the limits of the frequency range. In this method, 15 dB is subtracted from the HAIC gain and a horizontal line is drawn across the frequency response curve at this level. The points at which the line cuts the response curve represent the limits of the frequency response.

ANSI Standards, like British Standards, provide for measurements such as SSPL 90, full-on gain, and reference test gain. Some of the major differences between these standards are outlined in Table 7.1. ANSI also provides for a frequency range to be stated. This is obtained with the volume control at the reference test position. The output at 1 kHz, 1.6 kHz and 2.5 kHz is averaged and 20 dB subtracted. From the resulting figure, a straight horizontal line is drawn across the frequency response curve of the hearing aid. The two points at which this horizontal line intersects the frequency response represent the limits of the frequency range.

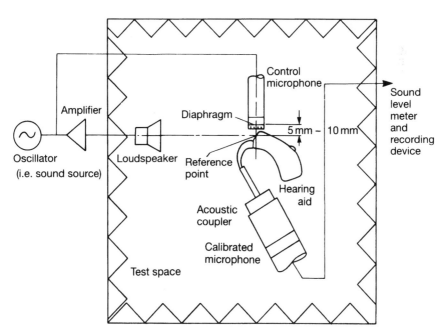

Fig. 7.10 A suggested arrangement for a postaural aid in a hearing aid test box.

7.5 MEASURING METHODS

7.5.1 THE TEST ENCLOSURE

The basic principle of hearing aid measurement is that with the controls of the aid suitably adjusted, an appropriate input signal is applied to the microphone of the aid and the output from the receiver is measured and analysed on a standardized device. Test methods and equipment have been standardized to permit accurate comparison.

The conditions under which the aids have been tested must be known and repeatable. The standards therefore use a specified test environment, which simulates essentially free-field conditions. This is a very quiet test space with sound absorbent walls and may be an anechoic chamber or a test box enclosure (Figure 7.10).

The test signal is generated by a sine wave oscillator and is fed to a loudspeaker within the test space. The hearing aid is accurately located at a determined test point, known as the reference point. The SPL in the test space is measured using a control microphone. The output of the hearing aid is transmitted through a standardized coupler to a calibrated microphone. The output of this microphone is recorded over the frequency range or examined for other characteristics, such as harmonic distortion.

7.5.2 COUPLERS IN USE

(a) Ear simulator (IEC 711)

The description of this coupler is contained in BS 6310 (1982).

An ear simulator is a device for measuring the output sound pressure of an earphone under well-defined loading conditions in a specified frequency range. Essentially it consists of:

- a principal cavity of specified volume;
- acoustic load networks;
- a calibrated microphone.

The location of the microphone is chosen so that the sound pressure at the microphone corresponds approximately to the sound pressure existing at the human eardrum. Therefore the ear simulator (Figure 7.11) is designed to simulate the average values of relevant acoustical characteristics of normal adult human ears.

The occluded ear simulator does not simulate the leakage between an earmould and a human ear canal (the effects of venting are not measured). Therefore the results obtained may deviate from real ear performance, especially at low frequencies. Moreover, large per-

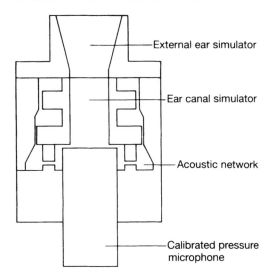

External ear simulator

Ear canal simulator

Acoustic network

Calibrated pressure microphone

Fig. 7.11 The basic parts of an occluded ear simulator.

formance variations among individual ears will occur and this should be borne in mind when employing results obtained with an ear simulator.

(b) Reference coupler (IEC 126)

The reference coupler is also known as an acoustic coupler and as a 2cc coupler (Figure 7.12).

The reference coupler is used as a simple and ready means of comparison of specifications and data on hearing aids. It does not allow the actual performance of a hearing aid on a person to be obtained.

The reference coupler is a cavity of predetermined shape and volume, which is used for 'the testing of earphones', in conjunction with a calibrated microphone adapted to measure the pressure developed within the cavity. It is described in BS 6111 (1981).

The SPL observed in an ear simulator compared to a 2cc coupler for any given input will show an increase of about 4 dB in the low frequencies, increasing gradually to about 15 dB higher at 10 kHz.

7.5.3 SIMULATED *IN SITU* WORKING CONDITIONS

Most methods for measuring the performance of hearing aids do not take into account the acoustical influence of the head and body of the wearer. However, methods which do so are relevant in the fitting of

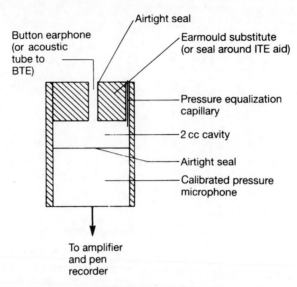

Fig. 7.12 The basic parts of a 2cc (reference) coupler.

hearing aids, since the results they produce relate to performance on the ear.

Real ear procedures (described in Chapter 10) can be used to provide *in situ* measurements for individual patients, but in order for *in situ* measurements to be quoted on a specification sheet, they must be standardized. This is achieved using a manikin, or anatomical model, to simulate the acoustical effects of a median adult wearer on the performance of a hearing aid.

The manikin simulates a head and torso and includes both an occluded ear simulator and an artificial pinna, or pinna simulator. Results using a manikin may be useful in assisting in hearing aid fitting, although care should still be taken when interpreting results. This is because results obtained from a manikin can be substantially different from those obtained on a real individual person, due to anatomical variations.

KEMAR is the Knowles Electronics Manikin for Acoustic Research. The BS and IEC Standards do not relate specifically to KEMAR. KEMAR was one of the first manikins available and uses a Zwislocki coupler, which was an early form of ear simulator.

The following parameters are considered essential for the evaluation of a hearing aid in simulated *in situ* conditions:

- full-on simulated insertion gain;
- insertion frequency response;

- directional characteristics;
- simulated *in situ* OSPL 90.

It may be noted that where simulated *in situ* conditions are used, the results may be presented in terms of *in situ* or insertion measures.

In situ measures describe the sound pressure level recorded in the real ear or in the ear simulator of the manikin. Thus, simulated *in situ* OSPL 90 refers to the maximum output recorded in the ear simulator of the manikin under the conditions specified in the relevant British Standard, BS 6083: Part 8 (1985).

Insertion measures consider the SPL in the ear, or ear simulator, of the manikin but under two different conditions – with and without a hearing aid. Insertion measures take account of the loss of natural amplification by making a simple comparison of the situation at the ear.

In situ measurements take no account of the loss of natural resonance that the hearing aid must overcome before it provides any advantage to the patient. Insertion gain represents the benefit on the ear. This appears lower than *in situ* gain because account is taken of the lost natural amplification (Figure 10.1).

Simulated *in situ* gain can be defined as the difference between the SPL in the ear simulator produced by the hearing aid and the reference input SPL.

Simulator insertion gain can be defined as the difference between the SPL in the ear simulator produced by the hearing aid and the SPL in the ear simulator with the hearing aid absent.

7.5.4 MEASUREMENT OF BONE VIBRATOR OUTPUT

Where a hearing aid employs a bone vibrator instead of an air conduction receiver a different method of measuring output must be used, and it becomes impractical to measure amplification directly in terms of acoustic gain. With bone conduction hearing aids, although the input is expressed in terms of sound pressure level, the output is described in terms of mechanical vibration. BS 6083: Part 9 (1986) defines a method of expressing the input/output ratio as an acoustic–mechanical sensitivity or force level. The mechanical coupler used to obtain this measurement is an artificial mastoid, or mastoid simulator (Figure 7.13), as specified in BS 4009 (1991).

The bone vibrator is secured to the artificial mastoid with a force of 2.5 newtons. The exact test assembly varies according to the type of bone conduction hearing aid. The standard provides for measurement of the force level in terms of gain and output across the frequency range 200 Hz to 5 kHz, and for the determination of distortion and internal noise.

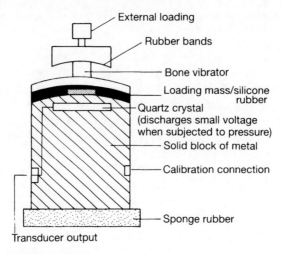

Fig. 7.13 An artificial mastoid.

7.6 POWER SOURCES

7.6.1 HEARING AID BATTERIES

A battery, or cell, is a package of chemically-stored energy that can be converted into electrical energy when the terminals are connected. Most batteries used in hearing aids are primary cells, that is they are used until the current is drained from them, at which point they are removed for disposal.

There are five sizes of batteries used in conventional hearing aids. Bodyworn aids employ the large 'penlite' cell which are identified by the IEC code R6 (BSI, 1987). The penlite cells used in bodyworn aids are generally the alkaline manganese type. Secondary, or rechargeable, cells may be used but these are mainly employed in radio hearing aids. Rechargeable batteries are of the nickel cadmium type.

Postaural and in-the-ear aids use button cells in one of four sizes, ranging from the largest, R44, commonly known as the 675 cell, to the smallest button cell, size 10, for which no IEC designation exists. The cells used in these aids are mercury or zinc air type.

7.6.2 BATTERY CHARACTERISTICS

There are certain characteristics of a battery that are important to hearing aid use. These include:

- The **capacity** of the battery is the current the battery can deliver over time, which is expressed in milliampere-hours.

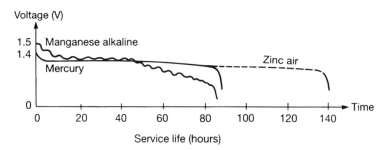

Fig. 7.14 Typical battery discharge characteristics on medium load (Duracell, 1990).

- The **nominal voltage** is a function of the chemistry of the battery and for new cells will be between 1.3 and 1.5 volts.
- The **discharge characteristic** is a graph that illustrates the change in the nominal voltage over time as the hearing aid is used (Figure 7.14).
- The **shelf life** is the period over which a battery can be stored without a significant loss in capacity. After a period of time, the capacity of the battery will reduce and this should not be allowed to exceed 10%.
- The **battery life** should be stated in the manufacturer's specification and will vary according to the capacity of the battery and the power requirement of the aid, which is mainly determined by the output stage of the amplifier.

Class A or single-ended amplifiers draw a constant average current drain from the battery, whether or not a signal is present (Figure 5.6). Once the aid is switched on a constant, or bias, current drain occurs. The introduction of the signal produces some variation about the bias value but the average drain remains constant. It is therefore simple to calculate battery life using the following formula:

$$\text{Battery life (hours)} = \frac{\text{Capacity (milliampere-hours)}}{\text{Current drain (milliamperes)}}$$

Class AB (more commonly, if incorrectly, termed class B), or 'push-pull' amplifiers draw very little current when there is no signal present (Figure 5.6). Battery drain increases as the output signal increases. Class AB, or B, amplifiers are more efficient but the variation in current drain makes it very difficult to predict the battery life with any degree of accuracy. The actual drain will vary with the signal level and with the volume setting. The life of the battery will be within a range that can be taken as the battery life with no signal present and the battery life with peak drain.

7.6.3 THE CHEMICAL COMPOSITION

(a) Alkaline manganese batteries

Alkaline manganese 'penlite' batteries used in hearing aids have a nominal voltage of 1.5 volts, a gradual discharge characteristic, a capacity of 2500 milliampere-hours and a shelf life of approximately 24 months.

The battery will recover slightly when left for a period without drain but, over time, it will gradually discharge. The gradual decay in use provides the adult user with some warning of the impending need to replace the battery, unlike the button cells which provide little or no warning. The quality of the output signal, however, also deteriorates as the battery runs down. The user can turn up the hearing aid to compensate for the battery decline but should certainly replace the battery if the sound quality is distorted.

Zinc carbon batteries are no longer used in hearing aids, due to a short shelf life and reduced capacity.

(b) Nickel cadmium batteries

Nickel cadmium batteries provide a steady discharge characteristic but have a short life. The batteries are normally recharged overnight. These are widely used in radio hearing aids.

(c) Mercuric oxide batteries

Mercury cells (mercuric oxide) have a shelf life of approximately 18 months and a nominal voltage of 1.3 volts. In use, after a slight initial reduction, the voltage remains constant for a long period. When the battery nears the end of its life the voltage decays very rapidly. The capacity of the cell depends upon its size; for example:

- size 675 has a capacity of 180 milliampere-hours;
- size 13 has a capacity of 90 milliampere-hours;
- size 312 has a capacity of 45 milliampere-hours.

Mercuric oxide batteries are extremely poisonous and should be kept out of the reach of children and animals. If a battery is swallowed medical attention must be sought promptly. The batteries should also be disposed of safely since they represent a source of pollution to the environment. The National Health Service collects all used batteries for return to the Department of Health for safe disposal.

(d) Zinc air batteries

Zinc air cells are supplied with an adhesive tab that must be removed to allow air to enter through small holes in the battery case. Once the tab is removed the battery will start to draw oxygen from the air and the life will start to reduce. Conventional cells contain both anode and cathode materials, but in zinc air batteries oxygen from the air reacts with a zinc anode via a thin catalytic cathode. This means the cell can contain much more anode material and that it can therefore produce more energy for the same volume of cell. The capacity of the cell is roughly double that of a mercury cell of the same size. The size 10 battery is so small it can only provide an acceptable life for hearing aids using zinc air design. The capacity of a size 10 zinc air battery is approximately 50 milliampere-hours.

Zinc air batteries have a shelf life of over two years and a very flat discharge profile. They are more 'environmentally friendly' than mercuric oxide batteries. However, if a high current drain is required, the battery may be unable to draw oxygen fast enough and a significant reduction in gain, or intermittency, may result. In these cases, usually where high gain and output or much filtering of the signal is required, mercury cells must be used.

7.6.4 RULES OF BATTERY STORAGE

1. Store in cool, dry conditions out of direct sunlight.
2. Rotate battery stock so that older batteries are used first.
3. Do not leave batteries in hearing aids if they are not in regular use.
4. Remove any white deposit on the contacts using a dry cloth.
5. Keep batteries away from fire.
6. Dispose of batteries safely.
7. Do not attempt to recharge primary cells.

7.7 THE NATIONAL HEALTH SERVICE PROVISION OF HEARING AIDS

7.7.1 THE NATIONAL HEALTH SERVICE RANGE OF HEARING AIDS

The National Health Service (NHS) provides hearing aids free of charge to all patients considered to obtain benefit from the use of an aid. In the majority of cases these fittings are monaural (one ear only) because of financial restrictions, but exceptions can be made if the life-style and hearing loss of the patient indicate the need for binaural hearing aids.

The NHS has a standard range of hearing aids, which includes a number of different models within certain series or strengths. These are made by various manufacturers but all conform to government specifications.

At present there are three behind-the-ear (BE) series:

1. The BE10 series provides moderate gain suitable for moderate hearing loss of up to 60 dBHL averaged over the essential speech frequencies from 500 Hz to 4 kHz. This series has five aids – the 16, 17, 18, 19 and 101 for issue and repair, and the 11 and 14 for repair only. The BE101 was introduced in 1992; it is the only NHS aid to incorporate AGC. It also uses a size 13 battery and is therefore significantly smaller than other NHS aids.
2. The BE30 series provides for moderate losses from 60 dBHL to 80 dBHL, and has the 34, 35 and 36 aids for issue and repair, and the 31, 32 and 33 for repair only. The BE36 was added to the range in 1992 and is suitable for hearing losses covered by both the BE30 and BE50 range. The BE36 is the only NHS aid to provide direct input, which enables it to be coupled directly to an FM radio system or other external audio source via an audio shoe and lead (Chapter 13). The specifications of the BE36 can be summarized as:

   • Standard MTO switch;
   • Direct audio input;
   • Continually variable tone and power controls;
   • Maximum full-on gain 65 dB (IEC 126);
   • .Maximum output 136 dB (IEC 126);
   • Choice of tone hooks.

3. The BE50 series is a higher powered series suitable for severe to profound hearing losses from 80 dBHL to 100 dBHL. This series has three aids, the 51, 52 and 53.

Bodyworn (BW) aids provide for severe and profoundly deaf patients and those who are unable to manipulate a small aid behind the ear. The BW61 is recommended for severe losses from 80 dBHL to 100 dBHL, the BW81 for severe to profoundly deaf patients. The Philips S1594, which has become available on the NHS, covers the same range as the BW81 but is smaller and lighter in weight and, from reactions from patients, gives greater clarity.

All these hearing aids are air conduction aids but a bone conductor on a headband can be fitted with the standard BW aids.

When selecting the appropriate hearing aid for patients, several factors need to be considered. The type and degree of the hearing loss, the size of the ear, the life-style of the patient and the position and ease of manipulation of the controls.

The earmould can have a considerable effect on the performance of a hearing aid, so care is therefore needed to select the most suitable mould for the hearing loss presented; also adjustments can be made to the aids to vary their frequency responses to match the hearing loss as closely as possible. However, if a patient's needs cannot be met from the standard range of NHS hearing aids other aids may be provided on the recommendation of the ENT consultant.

In general, the range is probably least suited to the needs of:

- very mild losses;
- unusual audiometric configurations;
- severe recruitment;
- children.

Policies vary throughout the country but in most regions children are provided with binaural hearing aids under the NHS. The facility of direct input (for radio hearing aids at school) can now be satisfied from the NHS range, but the BE36 will not be suitable for all children and commercial aids will still be required; for example, where a smaller aid is needed. However, when the child reaches the age of 18 and leaves school, funding for commercial aids is often no longer available.

7.7.2 OBTAINING AN NHS HEARING AID

A patient wishing to obtain an NHS hearing aid must first visit his or her doctor who will, if he or she considers it necessary, refer the patient to the ENT Department at the hospital. The patient will normally see the ENT consultant who will examine the patient's ears, take a case history and arrange for tests to be done to establish the type and degree of the hearing loss. An audiology technician will usually carry out these tests. The consultant will make the decision as to whether a hearing aid is indicated and appropriate, and which ear should be fitted. He or she may suggest which aid will be most suitable, but more commonly this is left to the discretion of the technician.

An ear impression is taken by the audiology technician for the earmould. When this has been made, a further appointment will be sent to the patient for the hearing aid fitting. The patient will be instructed in the use of the aid, how to insert the mould into the ear, its care and cleaning, the correct battery to use and how and when to replace it. The patient will also be informed of where they can obtain the batteries.

The degree of follow-up varies widely throughout the country depending on the resources available in individual hearing aid departments, but follow-up is desirable to meet the rehabilitative needs of the patients and to enable and encourage them to obtain the best possible use from their hearing aid.

Hearing aid departments also provide facilities for repair and servicing of aids and patients with bodyworn aids are able to obtain replacement cords and receivers. It is essential that patients are encouraged to visit the departments regularly to have their aids and moulds checked, the tubing replaced and the aid upgraded when necessary. All these services, and supplies of replacement batteries, are free of charge under the NHS.

7.8 SUMMARY

Hearing aids may be air or bone conduction systems. The performance of each aid is described in a standardized manner in a specification sheet. Various standards are available, but in the UK British Standards or their European equivalent (IEC) are most widely used. Characteristics presented in the specification include gain, maximum output, frequency response, distortion and internal noise. The measurements will show some variation depending on the coupler employed in the hearing aid test system. An ear simulator is generally used by manufacturers, while a 2cc coupler, which is a cheaper and simpler device, provides repeatable results for quality control on delivery.

A manikin may be used to simulate the results that would be obtained if a hearing aid was being worn by a median adult. Such results may be useful in hearing aid fitting but can be substantially different from some 'real life' clients due to anatomical variations.

Bone conduction hearing aids are coupled to an artificial mastoid and measurements are expressed in terms of mechanical vibration, instead of acoustic gain.

The batteries used in hearing aids vary in size and chemical composition. A number of characteristics are important to hearing aid use; these include the shelf life, the discharge characteristic and the battery life, which can be calculated from the formula:

$$\text{Battery life (hours)} = \frac{\text{Capacity (milliampere-hours)}}{\text{Current drain (milliamperes)}}$$

The NHS provides a standard range of bodyworn and behind-the-ear hearing aids. There are three series of behind-the-ear aids, the BE10, BE30 and BE50 series. Each comprises several different hearing aids, individually numbered, conforming to the required basic specification for the particular series. The BE10 series provides for moderate losses, the BE30 for moderate to severe losses, and the BE50 for severe to profound losses. NHS-provided hearing aids are supplied on loan without charge.

REFERENCES

ANSI (1987) *ANSI 5322: Specification for Hearing Aid Characteristics*, American National Standards Institute.

BSI (1981) *BS 6111: Specification for Reference Coupler for the Measurement of Hearing Aids using Earphones Coupled to the Ear by means of Ear Inserts*, British Standards Institution.

BSI (1982) *BS 6310: Specification for Occluded Ear Simulator for the Measurement of Earphones Coupled to the Ear by Ear Inserts*, British Standards Institution.

BSI (1984) *BS 6083: Part 0: Methods for Measurement of Electroacoustical Characteristics*, British Standards Institution.

BSI (1984) *BS 6083: Part 2: Methods for Measurement of Electroacoustical characteristics of Hearing Aids with Automatic Gain Control Circuits*, British Standards Institution.

BSI (1985) *BS 6083: Part 8: Methods for Measurement of the Performance Characteristics of Hearing Aids under Simulated* in situ *Working Conditions*, British Standards Institution.

BSI (1986) *BS 6083: Part 9: Methods for Measurement of Characteristics of Hearing Aids with Bone Vibrator Output*, British Standards Institution.

BSI (1987) *BS 397: Part 2: Primary Batteries. Specification Sheets*, British Standards Institution.

BSI (1988) *BS 6083: Part 10: Guide to Hearing Aid Standards*, British Standards Institution.

BSI (1991) *BS 4009: An Artificial Mastoid for the Calibration of Bone Vibrators used in Hearing Aids and Audiometers*, British Standards Institution.

Duracell (1990) *Guide for Designers*, Duracell, Crawley.

Pollack, M.C. (1988) *Amplification for the Hearing-Impaired*, 3rd edn, Grune & Stratton, Orlando.

Sullivan, R. (1989) Custom Canal and Concha Hearing Instruments: A Real Ear Comparison. *Hearing Instruments*, **40**(4), 29–9.

Upfold, L.J., May, A.E. and Battaglia, J.A. (1990) Hearing Aid Manipulation Skills in an Elderly Population: A Comparison of ITE, BTE and ITC Aids. *British Journal of Audiology*, **24**(5), 311–18.

FURTHER READING

BS 6083: Hearing aids:

(1984) Part 0: Methods for measurement of electroacoustical characteristics.

(1984) Part 1: Method for measurement of characteristics of hearing aids with induction pick-up coil input.

(1984) Part 2: Methods for measurement of electroacoustical characteristics of hearing aids with automatic gain control circuits.

(1984) Part 3: Methods for measurement of electroacoustical characteristics of hearing aid equipment not entirely worn on the listener.

(1981) Part 4: Specification for magnetic field strength in audio-frequency induction loops for hearing aid purposes.

(1984) Part 5: Specification for dimensions of the nipple and sealing device for insert earphones.

(1985) Part 6: Specification for characteristics of electrical input circuits for hearing aids.

(1985) Part 7: Methods for measurement of the performance characteristics of hearing aids for quality inspection on delivery.

(1985) Part 8: Methods for measurement of the performance characteristics of hearing aids under simulated *in situ* working conditions.

(1986) Part 9: Methods for measurement of characteristics of hearing aids with bone vibrator output.

(1988) Part 10: Guide to hearing aid standards.

(1984) Part 11: Specification for symbols and other markings on hearing aids and related equipment.

EverReady (1980) *Modern Portable Electricity*, EverReady Company, London.

Selection and fitting   8

8.1 THE CHOICE OF A HEARING AID SYSTEM

8.1.1 INTRODUCTION

The primary purpose and function of hearing aid systems is to enable hearing impaired people to make maximum use of their residual hearing area. A system should therefore provide maximum speech intelligibility, maximum useful information from other sounds, minimum interference from unwanted noise, and minimum distortion. The aim will normally be to provide amplified speech that is as clear and intelligible as possible, with the provision also of important background sounds, such as a ringing doorbell, or the sound of an approaching car. These environmental sounds are important not only as warnings, but also as providers of general information about our environment, which is important psychologically. Unfortunately, background noise can, and does, interfere with the speech signal and it can be difficult, or even impossible, for hearing impaired people to separate the sounds they want to hear, from those they do not. This is partly due to the defective hearing mechanism, which is especially notable where cochlear damage has been sustained, and partly to the restrictions inherent in a hearing aid.

A hearing aid system that will provide as little interference as possible from unwanted noise should be chosen. There are a number of features that can be selected or modified to minimize the problems, although the degree of success that can be achieved may be limited by the type of hearing loss. The hearing aid itself is a piece of man-made equipment and, however good, sound that is amplified and passed through the system will be distorted to some extent. A hearing aid with unacceptably high distortion should not be selected; this generally means no more than 10% in terms of total harmonic distortion (Tucker and Nolan, 1984).

The hearing aid fitting procedure includes the selection, 'fitting', evaluation and modification of a hearing aid system. Reliable audiometric information provides the starting point and information is required for threshold levels by air and bone conduction, most comfortable levels and uncomfortable loudness levels, across the appropriate frequency range (Chapter 6). The success of the fitting is dependent both on the reliable measurement of residual hearing and on an understanding of the electro-acoustic and other characteristics of hearing aids. It is also influenced by the effectiveness of the earmould. There are rules associated with the prescription and fitting of hearing aids. Although the amplification needs of the hearing impaired population remain not fully known, and the area of hearing aid fitting is one in which options, attitudes and traditions vary widely, the following questions may provide a starting point for selection:

- Is the fitting to be by air conduction or bone conduction?
- Is the fitting to be monaural or binaural?
- How much gain is needed?
- What maximum power output is required?
- Is there a need for automatic gain control?
- What are the required frequency response characteristics?
- What other facilities are needed?
- Is the aid acceptable to the client?

Client preference is an aspect of selection that should not be underestimated, for if a client does not accept the system, or if he or she cannot operate it with ease, its use will be seriously limited.

8.1.2 AIR CONDUCTION AND BONE CONDUCTION

Hearing aids can be obtained in the form of air conduction or bone conduction. Bone conduction aids are less efficient, require more power and have limited response capabilities; if bone conduction is necessary the choice will be extremely limited. Therefore, air conduction aids should be used whenever possible. Bone conduction fittings may have to be made because of certain conductive problems, for instance where there is a physical deformity, such as no pinna, a collapsed meatus, a tender post-operative condition, or where there is an active discharge from the ear. In such cases, there is often no real option.

If there is a choice, an air conduction fitting will normally be preferable for both sensorineural and conductive hearing losses. Occasionally there may be more benefit from a bone conduction hearing aid if there is a very severe conductive loss, caused by a gross obstruction or lesion in the middle ear, but it should never be assumed that bone conduction aids will necessarily provide the greater benefit. The efficiency of the coupling of an air conduction receiver to the meatus is greater than the mechanical coupling of a bone conduction vibrator to the mastoid, so that, in general terms, air conduction does not have to be as powerful as bone conduction to give the same effective output. It follows therefore that there is less risk of distortion in the output.

Air conduction hearing aids also provide other advantages. They are smaller and lighter, the frequency range is significantly wider than that of bone conduction, especially at the higher frequencies that are important to most hearing impaired people, and the response is also more readily and easily modified. Great benefit should not be expected from a bone conduction hearing aid if the hearing loss by bone conduction is much greater than 30 dB over 50% or more of the audiometric measurement points between 250 Hz and 5 kHz. Little gain is provided at frequencies beyond 5 kHz by a bone conduction aid and these aids are not helpful for sensorineural losses. In the case of mixed loss they will only be beneficial if the sensorineural element is not too great.

Three types of bone conduction aids, spectacle, postaural with headband, and bodyworn with cord and headband, are available; all employ a large, stiff receiver which must fit properly on the mastoid process and be under reasonable tension, or there will be a great tendency to mechanical and acoustic feedback.

In practice, the user's needs can generally be met more efficiently with air conduction than bone conduction hearing aids, and as air conduction can be applied equally well to a conductive as a sensorineural loss, air conduction hearing aids should be selected every time, unless there are strong medical contra-indications.

8.1.3 MONAURAL AND BINAURAL

A binaural hearing aid system consists of two complete hearing aids so that each ear is provided with its own separate microphone, amplifier and receiver. A system that provides sound to each ear, but which utilizes only one microphone, cannot supply all the benefits of true binaural hearing (Figure 8.1).

The benefit of binaural fitting, in suitable cases, greatly exceeds that of monaural, by providing more natural 'balanced' hearing with the advantages of:

- improved localization of the sound;
- improved sense of distance from the sound source;
- improved speech discrimination in noise;
- binaural summation;
- binaural frequency advantage;

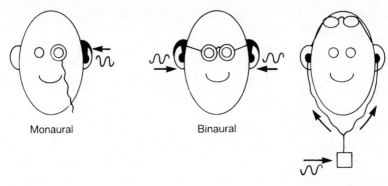

Monaural　　　　　　　　　Binaural

Pseudo-binaural

Fig. 8.1 Monaural, binaural and pseudo-binaural hearing aid fittings compared with spectacle fittings. The general public expects to have vision improved in both eyes, not only in one. Although hearing aids do not restore normal hearing in the same way as spectacles may restore normal vision, if both ears will benefit from amplification, two aids should be provided whenever practical.

- improved quality with less distortion;
- avoidance of abnormal headshadow effects;
- a subjective feeling of balanced hearing;
- masking for bilateral tinnitus;
- reduced likelihood of ever being without an aid;
- avoidance of auditory deprivation.

Small differences in the information arriving at each ear allow the listener to localize the sound source and to determine its distance away. The use of behind-the-ear and in-the-ear hearing aids permits full advantage to be taken of phase, time and intensity differences in the auditory signal arriving at each ear. These directional clues assist the brain in the selection of meaningful signals from competing background noise (Carhart, 1965). Sounds heard binaurally are also perceived as louder, usually by about 3 dB to 5 dB, than when heard monaurally, due to 'binaural summation' (Dermody and Byrne, 1975). Similarly, where each ear has a different response across the frequency range of the audiogram, the brain may be able to add this information together to provide a much improved pattern of sound for the listener. Problems produced by the 'headshadow effect', when hearing is only possible through one ear, are avoided by binaural hearing aid fitting (Figure 8.2).

The headshadow effect can be explained as follows. The head blocks the passage of any sound waves that have a shorter wavelength than the width of the head. The average head width is approximately 20 cm

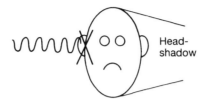

Fig. 8.2 The headshadow: the head blocks the passage of high frequency sound waves, preventing them from being heard on the other side. With a monaural loss, high frequencies from the deaf side will therefore tend not to reach the good ear.

and this means that the listener is at a great disadvantage, particularly with the high frequencies of speech if the sound source is on the same side as the poor ear. There is generally no significant attenuation below about 1.5 kHz, and the average attenuation that can be expected is:

1 dB at 250 Hz
2 dB at 500 Hz
3 dB at 1 kHz
6 dB at 2 kHz
10 dB at 4 kHz
25 dB at 6 kHz.

The higher the frequencies, the greater is the intensity difference between the two ears. With monaural hearing this creates problems that are heightened if background noise is present as this may mask the quieter high frequency sounds.

Wernick (1985) suggests that a sufficient body of research literature now exists for it to be reasonable to assume a binaural fitting advantage exists unless there is evidence to the contrary. This is of particular importance since it is sometimes difficult to demonstrate binaural advantage in the fitting process. Many clients report subjective improvement of sound quality and a feeling of balance especially after a period of rehabilitation. The use of two hearing aids has the very practical advantage that the client is not without a hearing aid if one is sent for repair, and two hearing aids may also offer some relief to sufferers of bilateral tinnitus. Children are routinely fitted binaurally and, in addition to all the aforementioned advantages, it is thought that binaural stimulation will avoid the effects of 'auditory deprivation', where permanent changes may occur in the auditory pathways when auditory signals are not received (Fisch, 1983). These changes may render the child less able to make good use of auditory information at a later stage. Auditory deprivation may also occur in adults that are aided monaurally, although some of the poorer performance at high presentation levels appears to be due to acclimatization (Gatehouse, 1990), that is the adult is used to listening to quiet signals in that ear, and therefore performs best at these levels, at least initially.

Not every user is able to benefit from binaural amplification and there are a few instances where binaural use results in a decrease in ability to understand speech, but the vast majority of clients can obtain some advantage. Binaural fitting should therefore always be tried, unless there is a reason not to do so. Reasons would include when a binaural fitting has previously been shown to be without adequate benefit, when there is a medical contra-indication, such as an active discharge from one ear, when there is poor manual dexterity on one side, or when a client refuses to accept binaural aids. Obviously, binaural hearing aids are also inappropriate if one ear is normal, or very near normal, or if one ear is 'dead'. In some cases, a CROS fitting may be more beneficial.

As a general rule, binaural fitting for adults with acquired hearing loss is likely to provide the greatest benefit when there is no more than a 20 dB gap between the two air conduction threshold curves at any frequency (Berger and Hagberg, 1989). The further apart the thresholds, the less benefit is likely to be achieved; but even grossly asymmetric ears can be successfully aided binaurally and a binaural fitting should only be dismissed if it is completely out of the question. Binaural fittings should be tried whenever possible, and the benefit assessed.

If a binaural fitting is not possible or desirable, the ear to be aided must be selected and this should always be the one that will yield most benefit. There is no hard and fast rule that can be applied to decide which ear this will be and there are a number of factors that must be considered. Speech tests are sometimes used with the aim of fitting whichever ear has the better speech discrimination. Tests do not always indicate an obvious advantage, and if one ear has been unused for some time, as is usually the case with asymmetric loss, it is difficult to estimate the value of the unused ear because the listener cannot immediately make use of the available information. Amplified sound fed to the better ear may at first appear more normal and easier to discriminate but, after a period of rehabilitation, the poorer ear might add to the information provided by the unaided response of the better ear.

As an alternative to speech discrimination testing, audiometric considerations may be used to decide which ear is likely to provide most benefit, and a rule of thumb often used is to fit the ear with the air conduction threshold which is nearest to 50 dBHL at 1 kHz. Other considerations may also affect the choice of ear to fit, and if there is a difference in uncomfortable loudness levels it may be preferable to fit the ear with the most normal uncomfortable loudness level (ULL) since this will provide a wider dynamic range. If unilateral tinnitus is present, fitting the ear with the tinnitus may provide some masking through the amplification of ambient noise; with certain medical conditions, such as physical abnormalities or recurrent discharge, it may be better, or necessary, to fit the ear without the problem.

The client's opinion and life-style should always be taken into consideration as there may be other reasons for having a preference for a certain ear. Where a client already uses a monaural hearing aid it is usually best to continue to use the same ear, since the user has already been rehabilitated to hearing on that side; this does not, of course, prohibit fitting the other ear, or introducing binaural use. Some types of employment pose particular hearing requirements; for instance, driving instructors need to hear in the right ear so they can hear their clients, while lorry drivers would probably be better with the hearing aid in their left ear so as to avoid excessive road noise, which could be picked up by a fitting in the road-side ear.

Clients may have a particular need or preference dictated by their life-style; this may be something as simple as the position of the television and chairs in the room and if audiometric and other considerations allow it client preference should be accepted. However, there are occasions where new users mistakenly believe that fitting the worst ear will most nearly correct their hearing defect whatever the loss, and counselling may be required to overcome an inappropriate belief of which ear will provide the most benefit.

8.1.4 CONTRALATERAL ROUTEING OF SIGNALS (CROS)

A unilaterally impaired person will have problems in hearing from the 'deaf' side and may need to turn the good ear towards the sound source. Such an impairment may cause particular hearing difficulty in background noise, hearing in groups, and in localization of sound. Slight differences in the time, frequency and phase of the signals reaching the left and right ears normally allow the selection of meaningful signals from competing noise and facilitate the localization of sound. Unilaterally impaired people manage well in most situations; they produce good free-field speech test results in quiet conditions, have no speech production problems, can use the telephone, hear the television, and have no noticeable difficulty in understanding. Their problems are very specific and, while the general public makes no allowance for unilateral loss, the hearing aid audiologist should not underestimate their difficulties. If medical intervention is not appropriate, hearing aid fitting may be helpful and there are two possible systems, a monaural fitting or a CROS system. The CROS system was developed to help the unilaterally impaired person to hear sounds from the deaf side. In cases where a binaural fitting is not possible

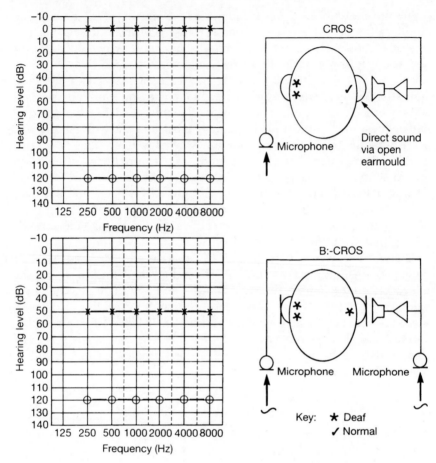

Fig. 8.3 Typical audiograms for CROS and Bi-CROS fittings.

because one ear is 'dead' or very severely impaired while the other has normal or at least much better hearing, a CROS or Bi-CROS system may be indicated (Figure 8.3).

In a CROS fitting, the signal is routed from the side of the 'dead' or severely impaired ear, to the normal or near normal ear, where it is received in addition to direct sound received in the good ear. A Bi-CROS fitting is used where the better ear is not normal and requires some amplification.

The acronym CROS stands for contralateral routeing of signals and Bi-CROS stands for bilateral contralateral routeing of signals. In a CROS system the microphone is placed at the poor ear, the receiver is placed at the good ear and an open earmould is fitted to allow direct entry of sound to the good ear, in addition to sound received from the deaf side. The Bi-CROS system is similar, except that it amplifies the sound received. Two microphones are employed, one at each ear, both connected to a single amplifier, which feeds the sound to the better but impaired ear, usually via a closed earmould. Venting is sometimes possible but this will depend on the degree of hearing loss, as venting will make the hearing aid system prone to acoustic feedback.

A CROS system offers some of the advantages of binaural fitting. It does not provide true binaural hearing but goes some way towards overcoming the problems of unilateral hearing, caused by the head-shadow effect. Some ability to localize sound can also be developed utilizing the differences in sound quality and time of arrival at each ear (Pollack, 1988). The unavoidable difference in the quality of sound received through the CROS system, compared with the natural sound received directly by the good ear, is particulary useful in this respect.

The option of fitting CROS and Bi-CROS hearing aids is not widely used. The advantages of fitting binaurally, even with gross asymmetry between the ears, is much more generally accepted and many ears that were previously viewed as unaidable are now shown to benefit from aiding. A CROS system can offer some of the advantages of binaural hearing to a client for whom only unilateral hearing would otherwise be possible, but it is a system that is physically more difficult to use and the client therefore needs to be highly motivated if the fitting is to be successful.

8.2 HEARING AID FITTING

8.2.1 THE REQUIREMENTS OF A ROOM FOR HEARING AID FITTING

A room for hearing aid fitting should provide a more realistic ambient noise level than the very quiet conditions required for audiometric testing. However, it is not desirable that a person using an aid for the first time should be exposed to loud sounds or a variety of different stimuli at once, as this could adversely affect the client's attitude to using hearing aids. This is an aspect of hearing aid fitting reflected in the rehabilitation of adults, where first time users are encouraged to build up their experience of aided sounds gradually from quiet situations to more complex noisy situations. In 1991 the British Society of Audiology proposed that a room used for the fitting of hearing aids should therefore have an ambient noise level not exceeding 40 dBA. The reverberation time should not exceed 500 milliseconds at 500 Hz to help avoid auditory confusion in the initial few minutes of hearing aid use. These acoustical requirements can normally be met by:

- siting the room away from obvious sources of noise, such as vehicular traffic, foot traffic (stairs, corridors), kitchens, toilets, doorbells, reception areas, etc.;

- having appropriate sound-excluding windows fitted and, if necessary, a second entrance door;
- ensuring that the floor is carpeted and the walls covered in absorbent material;
- ensuring that the seating is soft and the windows covered by heavy curtains;
- ensuring that the sound of any necessary ventilation equipment does not increase the overall ambient noise level.

8.2.2 THE FITTING PROCEDURE

(a) Gain

Whatever type of hearing aid system is selected the gain of the aid should be sufficient to give an acoustic output level that provides optimum speech discrimination and is centred on the user's most comfortable level. We are normally most interested in speech as the input signal and all methods of hearing aid selection and fitting seek to amplify speech so that it is delivered at a comfortable level for the hearing aid user. The speech signal changes rapidly in frequency, time and intensity. There is an intensity range of approximately 28 dB between the strongest and weakest components of speech. The average range of speech energy expressed in dBHL is sometimes drawn on the audiogram (Figure 8.4). This, which is known as the long-term average speech spectrum, indicates the normal average variation that occurs in

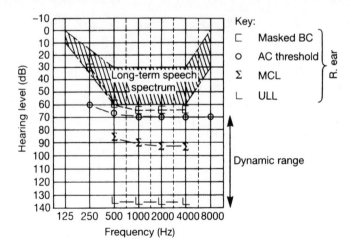

Fig. 8.4 An audiogram showing thresholds, MCL's and ULL's for the right ear. The gain of the hearing aid should be such that the output is centred on the user's most comfortable level (MCL). The maximum output should remain just below the user's uncomfortable loudness level (ULL).

conversational speech. It can be a very useful check on the benefit that may be expected from the amplification to be provided.

The amount of gain required by most hearing aid users is less than that which would appear to adjust the hearing thresholds to 'normal' levels, perhaps due to the effects of recruitment, where small increases in the objective intensity of a sound produce abnormally large increases in the subjective sensation of loudness. A client with a 60 dBHL hearing loss, for example, will neither require, nor be able to use, 60 dB of gain. Sensorineurally impaired people appear to require an amount of gain that is equivalent to about 50% of their hearing loss (Berger, Hagberg and Rane, 1980).

Several prescriptive procedures, each based on this 50% or 'half gain' rule, are now widely used to suggest the amount of gain the client needs with the volume control set for normal use. A hearing aid should generally be worn with the volume control about half-way on, which will usually provide about two-thirds of the possible gain. This allows the user some degree of control, to turn the aid up or down as circumstances dictate, and avoids the necessity to use the aid at full-on volume, where distortion is highest. However, hearing aids are often chosen from the full-on volume given in the specifications and it is therefore usual to estimate the full-on requirements. These can be approximated by multiplying the required user gain by 1.5, or by adding an amount of 'reserve gain', which is usually about 10 dB. A single figure of gain can be used for the purpose of choosing an aid that is 'in the right ball park', and the single figure most usually used is the amount of gain required at 1 kHz. This works well for reasonably 'flat' audiograms, but where there is a great difference between the frequency points it is usually preferable to determine the maximum amount of gain required in the region 500 Hz to 2 kHz on the audiogram. It should be noted that if a client has a very steeply sloping audiogram culminating in a severe to profound loss in the higher frequencies, the dynamic range at these frequencies is often too restricted to make full use of amplification and in this case the only practical solution may be partial correction of the hearing loss, in order to avoid discomfort, distortion and feedback. The position is very different for a client with conductive hearing problems. Since the inner ear has not sustained damage, recruitment is not present and the user will both need, and be able to cope with, increased gain.

There may also be some variation of the amount of gain required for those with very profound sensorineural loss. A client with a very profound loss may benefit from two-thirds gain, rather than only half, in order to receive speech at a more audible level (Libby, 1986). The use of a long-term average speech spectrum superimposed on the audiogram (Figure 8.4), will help to clarify whether the gain to be provided will amplify speech sufficiently to be audible. It is not unusual to have to provide a level of amplification that is at the bottom of the most comfortable area in order to achieve adequate hearing for more severe and profound losses. If the estimated gain is subtracted from the hearing threshold levels and placed on the audiogram, it will indicate the estimated aided threshold levels. The difference between the aided threshold levels and the lower limit of the speech spectrum will indicate the sensation level, or how much of the normal conversational speech signal the client would be likely to hear.

It is sometimes suggested that clients with a very mild loss require only one-third gain (Libby, 1986). From my own clinical observation, a starting point of insertion gain approximating to half the hearing loss for selection of a hearing aid works very satisfactorily for these clients as well, although less reserve gain may be required. It should be noted that the small in-the-canal aids, which are often used for very mild losses, appear to have a lower gain when tested using a 2cc coupler than when used on a real ear (Tate, 1990). When working with 2cc measurements rather than real ear gain, a one-third rule appears more appropriate.

Prescriptive formulae are designed to provide a practical method of estimating the appropriate gain for a given hearing loss, and they can provide a starting point for the fitting procedure. There are several prescriptive formulae that may be used. There is no consensus as to which formula may be most appropriate, but in almost every case the hearing aid audiologist should expect to have to 'fine tune' the hearing aid at the evaluation stage.

Most formulae present the gain requirements in terms of functional gain or insertion gain. Functional gain is the gain of the hearing aid on the ear and may be taken as the difference between aided and unaided hearing thresholds. Insertion gain is also a measure of functional gain, but it is less confusing to consider it separately.

Insertion gain is the difference between the sound pressure level aided and unaided, measured with a probe microphone near the eardrum. It is the true or effective gain of the system and takes into account the natural amplifying effect of the normal open ear, which is lost or altered when the ear is blocked with the hearing aid. Hearing aid specification sheets do not always give insertion gain but, where it is not stated as such, insertion gain can be derived by subtracting the open ear response from the *in situ* gain or KEMAR gain. Similarly, insertion gain can be approximately established from 2cc measures of gain by adding a correction factor, which will vary according to the type of aid but at 1 kHz is approximately 3 dB for a behind-the-ear aid and 4 dB for an in-the-ear aid.

The original half gain rule dates back to at least 1944, when Lybarger is said to have applied for a patent that specified an amplification range between one-third and two-thirds, although the patent was denied on legal grounds. In 1953, Lybarger published his fitting procedure in *The Basic Manual for Fitting Radioear Hearing Aids*, and in 1957 he presented the procedure at the American Speech and Hearing Association convention. The formula still works well and is readily understandable in that it takes account of binaural advantage and of the need for increased gain with conductive losses:

$$\text{Required operating gain} = \frac{\text{AC Loss}}{2} + \frac{\text{AC} - \text{BC}}{4} + 5\,\text{dB}$$

This provided a single figure of gain, which is often all that is required as a starting point, when the gain is to be considered together with the shape of the frequency response indicated from the audiogram. The constant of $+5\,\text{dB}$ was adjusted to a figure of $-10\,\text{dB}$ if the fitting was to be binaural, and finally $15\,\text{dB}$ of reserve gain was added, although I have found the figure of $15\,\text{dB}$, both for binaural advantage and for reserve gain, to be generally more than is required.

(b) Frequency response

The shape of the frequency response curve must be suitable for the frequency characteristics of the hearing loss. Most clients with mild to severe hearing losses require a response from their hearing aids that 'mirrors' the shape of the audiogram in as much as it provides most gain where the hearing loss is greatest. If a simple half gain rule is adopted, taking 50% of the hearing loss, each frequency point will automatically provide a frequency response characteristic which should be near to that required, although the gain at 500 Hz and below has often to be further reduced in order that the higher frequencies may be perceived more clearly. Hearing aids may be obtained that provide adjustable tone controls (section 5.3).

Where a single figure of gain is used to select possible hearing aids, whether this be from a single frequency point, usually 1 kHz, or from an average across the midfrequency range, usually 500 Hz to 2 kHz, the slope of the audiogram must be further considered to ensure that the frequency characteristics of the aid are suitable across the amplification range.

It is usual to provide less gain in the low frequency region (section 5.3.2), except for clients with more severe and profound hearing losses who may rely upon amplification of this region, and, where low frequency hearing is near normal, venting may be used to further reduce the low frequency gain. The degree of low frequency reduction suggested by the various formulae varies somewhat. A reduction of 5 dB at

500 Hz is recommended by McCandless and Lyregaard (1983) in the 'POGO' prescription of gain and output for hearing aids, whereas Libby (1986), in the 'one-third–two-thirds gain' rule, provides for slightly less low frequency reduction: 3 dB at 500 Hz and only 5 dB at 250 Hz. This prescription provides for the use of the same correction factors with gain of one-third, half, or two-thirds, respectively, for mild, moderate, and severe to profound hearing losses. Libby also suggests that where the hearing loss is precipitously falling, a 'ski-slope' type audiogram, patients usually prefer a gain of about one-third, rather than half of the hearing loss. The formula presented by Berger (1988) is yet another variation of the half gain rule, but one which provides for slightly more than half gain in the midfrequency region (Table 8.1).

High frequency amplification is important for clarity and intelligibility but over-amplification may produce an aid that sounds 'tinny' and too quiet and which is also prone to acoustic feedback. Clients who are new to hearing aids, particularly those who have been in need of amplification for some while, are sometimes unable, initially, to adjust to a level of high frequency amplification that should be beneficial to them. In such cases it is often possible to increase the high frequency amplification after a period of rehabilitation.

(c) Maximum output

The maximum power output must be selected and, if necessary, further set by the hearing aid audiologist so that the saturation sound pressure level (SSPL) is not capable of frequently exceeding the user's uncomfortable loudness level (ULL).

All hearing aids have a limit to the maximum output they are able to provide and in many hearing aids with linear amplification this limit is

Table 8.1 Examples of variation in prescription of insertion gain using different formulae

Frequency (Hz)	Predicted insertion gain (dB)		
	Libby	POGO	Berger
250	(HTL* ÷ 2) − 5	(HTL ÷ 2) − 10	HTL ÷ 2
500	(HTL ÷ 2) − 3	(HTL ÷ 2) − 5	HTL ÷ 2
1 k	HTL ÷ 2	HTL ÷ 2	HTL ÷ 1.6
2 k	HTL ÷ 2	HTL ÷ 2	HTL ÷ 1.5
3 k	HTL ÷ 2	HTL ÷ 2	HTL ÷ 1.7
4 k	HTL ÷ 2	HTL ÷ 2	HTL ÷ 1.9
6 k	(HTL ÷ 2) − 5	HTL ÷ 2	HTL ÷ 2

*HTL = hearing threshold level

Table 8.2 Factors that can be added to dBHL to convert thresholds to dBSPL (Based on recommended reference equivalent threshold sound pressure levels in a coupler in accordance with BS 2497: Part 5 (1988))

500 Hz	1 kHz	2 kHz	4 kHz
11.5	7	9	9.5

in the region of 120 dBSPL, although it can be higher. The maximum output of the aid can often be reduced from its natural limit using peak clipping. The ULL may be used to guide the setting of the maximum output, which should be as high as possible while remaining at least 5 dB below the ULL. This is not as straightforward as it would at first appear. The ULL in dBHL provides only a rough guide to the maximum output setting in dBSPL that will be required by the user in everyday life. The ULL on the audiogram is recorded in dBHL, while the maximum output of the hearing aid is in dBSPL. Conversion factors can be added to dBHL thresholds to provide an approximation to dBSPL (Table 8.2).

Also, ULL's from the audiogram have been obtained using pure tones while in everyday situations hearing aid users are hearing complex sounds, including speech, for which improved ULL thresholds would be obtained. Therefore, when estimating the maximum output from the ULL on the audiogram, a figure greater than the ULL shown on the audiogram can be assumed, although opinions vary on the degree of difference that can be added, and such correction factors range from 4 dB to 20 dB (McCandless and Lyregaard, 1983).

The use of different couplers in the measurement of the output of the hearing aid also creates a significant variation. The maximum output of the hearing aid in dBSPL will appear higher with ear simulator or *in situ* data than the same hearing aid measured using a 2cc coupler. It would therefore appear fairly logical to use a higher conversion factor to add to the ULL from the audiogram when considering *in situ* data, and in clinical practice I have found that an addition of 10 dB to 20 dB has generally been possible without discomfort, whereas an addition of only 5 dB to 10 dB is more usual when working from 2cc data. Adjustment may also be necessary because the instructions given in administering the subjective ULL test may influence the discomfort levels recorded.

Whatever method is employed to select the maximum output to be used, it must always be evaluated when the hearing aid is worn by the client. The maximum output of an aid should never be set such that it causes discomfort in everyday use. Where a single figure is required for the maximum output, this can be obtained either by using the 1 kHz reading or by averaging, usually over the frequencies 500 Hz to 2 kHz.

(d) Automatic gain control (AGC)

The maximum output should ideally be set at least 30 dB above threshold as this will allow a range between threshold and discomfort that is sufficient to appreciate the different intensity levels in the speech signal. However, in some instances of very restricted dynamic range, an aid set such that the maximum output is 5 dB below discomfort cannot provide this difference. Amplification is then only likely to be successful if automatic gain control is utilized.

Some form of automatic gain control, which is also known as compression, may be needed to deal with a severe recruitment problem, and the choice between linear amplification and the use of compression is usually dependent on the dynamic range of the user, although some audiologists consider that all sensorineurally impaired users would benefit from compression with a high threshold or 'kneepoint' (Dillon, 1988). The choice between compression and peak clipping will take account of both the audiogram and the client's needs and situation.

Peak clipping provides an excellent and instantaneous safeguard against uncomfortably loud sounds, but with severe recruitment a small dynamic range will mean that, if peak clipping alone is used to limit the output, weak sounds will not be heard while intense sounds will be too loud (Figure 5.13). Automatic gain control compresses the signal within the available dynamic range. This avoids high distortion, which would occur with frequent peak clipping, yet retains the important information content of the signal. Comfort levels can provide a most useful guide to the likely benefit to be derived from automatic gain control and, as a general rule, if the difference between the MCL (most comfortable level) and the ULL is 25 dB or more, no compression is required. With a difference of less than 20 dB, compression will be beneficial. With a difference of less than 15 dB, compression is often essential. The AGC kneepoint should be set as high as possible to maintain the user's maximum dynamic range. Peak clipping offers sufficient protection for most hearing aid users against loud environmental sounds. Peak clipping only affects intense sounds and therefore does not generally affect speech intelligibility. Although peak clipping does cause distortion, this usually occurs with environmental sounds, such as traffic noise, where distortion is largely irrelevant. But this is not always the case and, for example, lovers of loud music may prefer output compression to reduce the distortion that would occur with peak clipping alone. On the other hand, where a very restricted dynamic range means that amplified voices are likely to cause discomfort, input compression will be considered an advantage for some patients.

Whichever method of output limiting is selected, it is essential that uncomfortable loudness levels are an accurate measure of discomfort rather than unpleasantness. If not, too much limiting may be employed, resulting in an unnecessary restriction of the client's dynamic range.

(e) Multichannel hearing aids

Multichannel hearing aids attempt to match the needs of the user more closely by treating different frequency bands or channels separately to produce a complex frequency response, with the aim of providing a precise prescription fitting. If the audiogram shape varies widely in the different frequency regions, or if the configuration is unusual, it may be helpful to use a twin or multichannel system. However, such systems do not always result in the anticipated extra benefit, perhaps because of the problems of poor sound perception due to cochlear damage.

8.3 SUMMARY

Effective amplification is vital for the rehabilitation of the hearing impaired. Hearing aid fitting is a mixture of art and science – a challenge to the skills of the hearing aid audiologist. The overall aim of the fitting is to provide an amplified signal that will allow maximum benefit to be gained from the residual hearing area. Hearing aids are selected according to the medical, audiological and other needs of the individual.

The basic priorities for the initial prescription of hearing aid characteristics can be summarized as the provision of:

1. the correct amount of gain, which is usually approximately equal to half the hearing loss by air conduction;
2. a maximum output that is not higher than the genuine ULL;
3. a frequency response that relates to the slope of the audiogram, without over-amplifying the low frequencies.

The aid selected should ideally be sufficiently flexible to allow modifications. These may be required especially in respect of the gain, frequency and maximum output.

REFERENCES

Berger, K.W. (1988) A Hearing Aid Fitting Method. *Audiology in Practice*, **5**, 1.
Berger, K.W. and Hagberg, E.N. (1989) An Examination of Binaural Selection Criteria. *Hearing Instruments*, **40**(9), 32, 44–6.

Berger, K.W., Hagberg, E.N. and Rane, R.L. (1980) A Re-examination of the One-Half Gain Rule. *Ear and Hearing*, **1**, 223–5.

British Society of Audiology (1991) *Proposals for Recommendations for a Room for Hearing Aid Fitting*, British Society of Audiology, Reading.

British Standards Institution (1988) *BS 2497: Part 5: Standard Reference Zero for the Calibration of Pure-Tone Air Conduction Audiometers*, British Standards Institution.

Carhart, R. (1965) Monaural and Binaural Discrimination against Competing Sentences. *International Audiology*, **4**, 5–10.

Dermody, P. and Byrne, D. (1975) Loudness Summation with Binaural Hearing Aids. *Hearing Instruments*, **26**, 22–3.

Dillon, H. (1988) Compression in Hearing Aids, in *Handbook of Hearing Aid Amplification*, Volume 1 (ed. R. Sandlin), College-Hill, Boston.

Fisch, L. (1983) Integrated Development and Maturation of the Hearing System. *British Journal of Audiology*, **17**, 137–54.

Gatehouse, S. (1990) Acclimatisation and Auditory Deprivation as Explanations for Changes in Speech Identification Abilities in Hearing Aid Users. *Proceedings of the Institute of Acoustics*, **12**(10), 31–7.

Libby, R. (1986) *The Insertion Gain Hearing Aid Selection Guide*. Hearing Instruments, **37**(3), 27–8.

McCandless, G. and Lyregaard, P. (1983) Prescription of Gain and Output (POGO) for Hearing Aids. *Hearing Instruments*, **34**(1), 16–21.

Pollack, M. (1988) *Amplification for the Hearing-Impaired*, 3rd edn, Grune and Stratton, Orlando.

Tate, M. (1990) The Application of Real Ear Probe Tube Measurements to Hearing Aid Fitting. *Acoustics Letters*, **14**(91), 1–6.

Tucker, I. and Nolan, M. (1984) *Educational Audiology*, Croom Helm, London.

Wernick, J.S. (1985) Use of Hearing Aids. *Handbook of Clinical Audiology*, 3rd edn, (ed. J. Katz), Williams and Wilkins, Baltimore, pp. 911–35.

FURTHER READING

Byrne, D. (1987) Hearing Aid Selection Formulae: Same or Different? *Hearing Instruments*, **38**(1), 5–11.

Pollack, M. (1988) *Amplification for the Hearing-Impaired*, 3rd edn, Grune & Stratton, Orlando.

Sandlin, R. (1988) *Handbook of Hearing Aid Amplification*, Volume 1, College-Hill, Boston.

Earmoulds 9

9.1 MAKING THE IMPRESSION

9.1.1 INTRODUCTION

The purpose of an earmould is to secure the aid to the ear and convey sound into the ear canal. The mould may also have a significant effect on the frequency response of the aid.

An earmould is the reverse duplication of the ear, obtained by taking an impression. The features of the impression are named after the parts of the pinna to which they relate, except that the helix is divided into the ball, waist and fan (Figure 9.1).

The taking of an impression is a vitally important part of the hearing aid fitting procedure and one that can make the difference between success and failure, for if the impression does not accurately reflect the pinna contours and the meatal projection, the quality of the system in terms of comfort and acoustic performance may be adversely affected.

9.1.2 IMPRESSION MATERIALS

Silicone-based materials are recommended for the taking of ear impressions (Nolan and Combe, 1985). There are two basic types currently available; condensation reaction silicone and addition cured silicone, and the choice will depend upon the requirements. Ideally, impression materials for making earmoulds should be easy to work with, including having suitable flow properties, and they should provide an accurate impression, which will be flexible but of sufficient mechanical strength not to deform or tear easily. They should not have undesirable side effects, such as producing heat, and they should remain stable over time.

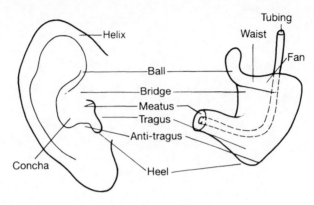

Fig. 9.1 The features of an earmould in relation to the pinna.

(a) Condensation reaction silicone

Condensation reaction silicone is currently the most widely used material. This cures by a condensation polymerization reaction, in which alcohol is produced in by-products, which evaporate. A small amount of shrinkage, accompanied by a weight loss of about 1%, results within the first 48 hours (Tucker and Nolan, 1984). This represents a great advance over acrylics, which are unstable and shrink about 6%, used prior to the introduction of silicone materials. However, even the small degree of shrinkage encountered with condensation reaction silicone can create a problem where a tight fitting earmould is required, namely where gain of over 50 dB is required, and for all children, especially during periods of rapid growth.

Condensation reaction silicone is not particularly easy to mix since the ratio of base to hardener is imprecise. Use of inadequate hardener can result in very slow curing, while too much can result in the material hardening before the impression has been completed. This material is considerably less expensive than its addition cured counterpart, provides a reasonably short setting time and results in a relatively elastic impression that travels well. This impression material is satisfactory for earmoulds where a tight fit is not vital, but is less satisfactory for high gain requirements or for children.

(b) Addition cured silicone

Addition cured silicone has two major advantages over condensation reaction silicones: improved dimensional stability; and ease of measuring the base and hardener mix. This material has no measurable shrinkage and is therefore able to produce very precise ear impressions.

It is mixed using equal parts of base and hardener, which is fairly easy to estimate or which can be achieved accurately using measuring syringes. It is considerably slower in setting than condensation reaction silicone and it is also more expensive, although this is a minor disadvantage in comparison with the advantages where precision is required. The set impressions are elastic and do not recover well from deformation, particularly in the early stages of curing; they should therefore be removed from the ear with great care, using a gentle rocking motion to avoid tearing.

If both addition cured and condensation reaction silicones are used, separate syringes must be kept for each material, as addition cured silicone is easily affected by contamination.

When packaging, ideally the ear impression should be glued by its base to a rigid box and not surrounded by packaging material. Paperwork should be placed outside the box. The use of pins to affix impressions to the box is no longer acceptable.

9.1.3 EAR IMPRESSION EQUIPMENT

The equipment necessary for taking an impression should be laid out on a clean surface; a clean white towel is generally preferred for this purpose. The following items are required:

- an otoscope with batteries to provide good illumination;
- at least three sizes of specula, in sterilizing solution or another suitable sterilizing environment;
- tweezers to remove the specula from the sterilizing solution;
- paper tissues to dry the specula;
- suitable impression material;
- an impression syringe;
- foam meatal blocks in three sizes;
- an earlight;
- a clean towel to place over the client's shoulder to protect clothing;
- scissors (round-nosed) for trimming very excessive meatal hair and for trimming or 'pruning' foam meatal blocks;
- lubricant (such as petroleum jelly) for smoothing down excessive meatal hair or remaining hair stubble after trimming.

9.1.4 THE EAR EXAMINATION

A thorough examination of the outer ear should always precede impression-taking (Chapter 6) to check for abnormalities that could necessitate referral to a medical practitioner, and to note any irregularities that might affect the procedure.

- Excessive wax may cause a conductive loss if the meatus is completely blocked. The impression procedure would be likely to further compress the wax and the client should therefore be referred to a medically-qualified person for its removal before the impression is made.
- The condition of the skin lining should be healthy and there should be no discharge, otherwise appropriate medical treatment is required prior to hearing aid fitting.
- Irregularities in the shape of the pinna or the meatus should be noted and care taken to ensure the impression indicates any relevant abnormalities. Any malformations that might be considered to be errors in the impression should be noted for the earmould manufacturer.
- Where there has been previous surgery, such as mastoidectomy, great care should be taken in the placement of the meatal block. A mastoidectomy involves the removal of diseased bone from behind the pinna, and this may affect the shape of the middle ear, including enlarging the external auditory meatus. In such a case particular care must be taken to ensure the impression material does not reach the wider parts, from which removal of the set material could be extremely difficult and might necessitate hospital treatment. The meatal block must be sufficiently large and placed with care, and syringing must be slow and careful, to avoid moving the block further down the meatus. In some extreme cases, the impression procedure could place the client at risk and should not be undertaken.
- The condition of the tympanic membrane should be noted and special care taken if the membrane is scarred, as scar tissue is weak and may be perforated, or if the ear is already perforated, since air pressure into the middle ear may cause dizziness. Care should be taken in positioning the foam block, slowly injecting the impression material into the ear and, when set, in very slowly removing the impression, so breaking the airtight seal with the ear very gradually.

9.1.5 THE EAR IMPRESSION TECHNIQUE

1. The client should be provided with a brief explanation of the technique to be employed, and should be made aware that there may be a feeling of fullness experienced in the ear. The mouth should be kept in the normal, naturally closed position and there should be no talking or jaw movement, other than swallowing to relieve the feeling of pressure, until the impression is set.
2. A towel or tissue should be placed over the client's shoulder and a suitably sized foam block should be selected, such that it will completely fill the meatus but without causing undue pressure. If

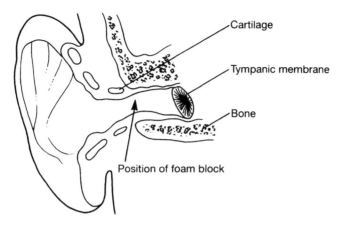

Fig. 9.2 Placement of the foam block when taking an impression. The block should be positioned just beyond the second bend, at the junction between the bone and the cartilage.

the client has a very small ear canal the foam block may be 'pruned' or 'tapered' with scissors to fit. The cotton threads should be knotted to ensure these cannot be accidentally removed, and the block should be gently inserted into the ear canal. Ear impressions should be taken from a sitting or kneeling position, so that the client's ear is at, or above, eye level. A hand should be held against the client's head to prevent discomfort if the client moves and the earlight should be used to position the block just beyond the second bend (Figure 9.2) at the junction between bone and cartilage, which is approximately half-way down the meatus. Sufficient depth in the meatus is important to provide an accurate indication of the angle of the bends of the meatus, in order that the mould-maker can place the output tube at the required angle to direct sound to the tympanic membrane and not towards the canal wall.

3. If spectacles or ear-rings are normally worn, these should not be removed and if the impression is being taken to produce an earmould for a behind-the-ear hearing aid, the aid should be placed on the pinna until the impression is set. If the ear is especially hairy a small amount of petroleum jelly can be applied to the hair to prevent it adhering to the set impression. Excessive hair can be carefully trimmed with scissors if the client gives permission, but this is only rarely necessary.

4. The impression material should be mixed quickly but thoroughly, and placed in the syringe. The plunger should be depressed so that material begins to flow out of the nozzle, thus expelling any air. The syringe should be positioned as near as possible to the foam block

and the material should be syringed steadily into the ear. When it begins to flow out of the meatus, the syringe should be moved to fill the concha, but with the nozzle always remaining slightly embedded in the material. When the concha has been partially filled, the helix should be filled, returning to the concha until it is completely filled. The concha should be filled sufficiently to indicate its depth but not to the extent that the impression begins to sag. The impression should not normally be pressed or smoothed off as this may distort it.

5. The impression material should be allowed to set until no mark is left if a finger-nail is lightly drawn across it. The impression may stretch if it is removed before it has fully set.
6. The set impression should be eased slowly from the ear, lifting the helix out first and then pulling gently at the base, or using a gentle rocking motion, in such a way as to avoid causing discomfort to the client or distortion of the impression.
7. The impression should not be trimmed but can be marked to indicate requirements, and should be carefully checked for accuracy before sending to the manufacturers.
8. The ear should be examined with an otoscope to ensure that all the impression material and the foam block have been removed, and the client should be offered a tissue to wipe the ear, which may be greasy.
9. The ear impression should be packaged carefully for transit, preferably glued to the base of a rigid box, and sent with its accompanying paperwork to specify the type of earmould and the material required.

9.2 EARMOULDS

9.2.1 EARMOULD MATERIALS

There are a number of materials available for the manufacture of earmoulds, and the selection will depend on the requirements necessary for the mould. Every client wants an earmould that will fit well and be comfortable, easy to insert and remove, easy to clean, of acceptable appearance and that will not cause acoustic feedback (whistling). There is no one ideal; each available type has its own advantages and disadvantages.

Hard acrylic is the most widely used material since it is an attractive product that is non-toxic, easy to clean, easy to work and can be produced in any configuration. It is not flexible and generally does not provide a sufficiently good acoustic seal for hearing aids with high gain, over approximately 50 dB. Soft acrylic is still a fairly hard material, but provides a more efficient acoustic seal and has a little more flexibility, which is often more comfortable and may also be advantageous for a client whose jaw moves to a greater than average extent. Soft acrylic is porous, not as easy to clean, and is stained by ear wax. It is a material that can be used on its own or as a soft tip in conjunction with a hard acrylic bowl.

There are a number of true soft or 'all soft' materials available, which include vinyl and silicone products. These provide an improved acoustic seal and are more comfortable. They may be recommended for children as they offer more protection if the child is hit on the ear. Soft materials cannot be produced in skeleton form as they lack the required strength and rigidity. They are difficult to modify and to retube, and they need retubing at frequent intervals, ideally as often as every two months, because the tubing tends to collapse within the earmould. They are also porous and more difficult to clean, and have a shorter life as they tend to split.

Soft materials, especially silicone, may be used in the manufacture of non-allergenic moulds, where these are required. True allergenic reactions to the materials used are rare and, more frequently, the irritation is due to the use of colourants or to oversized or rough earmoulds.

9.2.2 EARMOULD TYPES

The earmould type will be selected (Figure 9.3) first according to whether the hearing aid is of the bodyworn, behind-the-ear, or in-the-ear type. A bodyworn aid requires a solid mould with a ring and clip fitting to accommodate the external receiver. Such a mould is usually supplied with a full helix to ensure that the extra weight of the receiver does not pull the mould out of the ear. It can be ordered in hard or soft materials and can be supplied with a wire to hook over the top of the pinna for further security if necessary. The style that can be selected for behind-the-ear aids is much wider and includes all those listed below. The earmould or shell of an in-the-ear aid contains the battery and workings of the aid, which restricts its size, but it can be produced as full shell, half shell, canal or helix fitting.

- A full shell completely fills the concha and can provide a good acoustic seal for high gain. It can be obtained with or without a full helix, which improves retention in the ear but may not be comfortable. The full shell is the most common style for in-the-ear hearing aids.
- A skeleton mould or invisimould is similar to the full shell but the centre of the concha portion is removed making the mould less conspicuous while remaining secure.

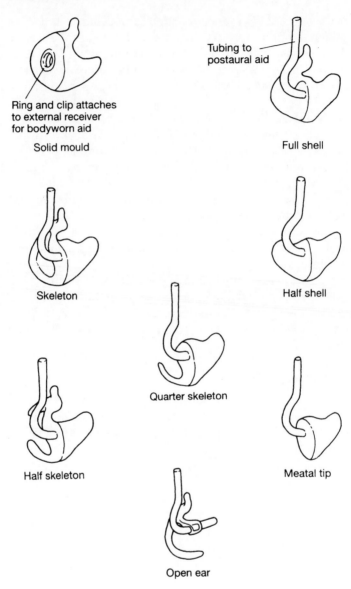

Fig. 9.3 Earmould types. (After Hearing Aid Audiology Group (1994).)

- Half-skeleton and quarter-skeleton moulds are variations of the skeleton mould in which part, or most, respectively, of the outer perimeter is removed, for comfort, ease of insertion or cosmetic purposes.
- A canal or meatal tip provides a less good acoustic seal and is less

secure in the ear, but is a very popular fitting because it is easy to insert and very inconspicuous.

- An open canal or CROS mould has no meatus and is usually a skeleton fitting, but it may be a full concha, to hold the tube into the meatus without causing occlusion.
- A helix in-the-ear aid provides an open canal fitting, in which the components of the aid are contained in the helix portion of the shell.

9.2.3 MODIFICATION OF HEARING AID PERFORMANCE

Modifications to the performance of a hearing aid may be made electronically and acoustically. Some hearing aids provide a number of electronic controls with which the hearing aid audiologist can adjust and modify the hearing aid's performance (section 5.3).

Acoustic modifications (Figure 9.4) are those that occur beyond the receiver, that is in the elbow or earhook, the tubing and the earmould, which together are sometimes referred to as 'the earmould plumbing'. These modifications may take the form of alterations to the tubing length or diameter, or to the length of the meatal projection, the addition of filters in the sound path and venting the earmould.

(a) Tubing modifications

The tubing affects the frequency response of the aid due to resonance (Chapter 1), which creates peaks in the sound output at certain frequencies. These frequencies are primarily dictated by the internal diameter of the tubing. The tubing length has some effect but is very difficult to adjust, as it is fixed by the size of the ear and the location of the hearing aid. The internal diameter of tubing can be readily used as a means of shifting the frequency emphasis. Decreasing the tubing diameter will lower the frequency emphasis, by lowering the frequency of the first resonant peak and reducing the mid- and high frequency

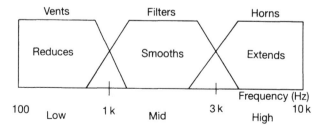

Fig. 9.4 The effect of various acoustic modifications. Venting affects the low frequency region, filters smooth peaks in the response, and horns extend the high frequency amplification.

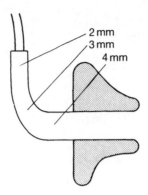

Fig. 9.5 A Libby horn.

gain and output. Conventional fittings use constant bore tubing, but it is possible to increase the diameter of the tube towards the ear canal to produce a significant improvement in high frequency response. This increase in high frequency, which is due to a quarter wave resonance, is known as a horn effect (Figure 9.5); a horn that provides a 4 mm final diameter will enhance the response above 3 kHz by about 10 dB, and extend the frequency limit, usually to about 8 kHz. A 3 mm horn can provide a similar enhancement, but only up to about 6 kHz. Increasing the high frequency response in this way may be very advantageous for some clients with high frequency hearing loss and, conversely, a tapered or reverse-horn arrangement, in which the diameter of the last section is reduced, may be used to attenuate the high frequencies, which may be helpful for some low frequency hearing losses. Where a higher frequency response is required from an in-the-ear hearing aid, some improvement may be achieved by increasing the diameter of the sound bore by 'belling' the end of the meatal projection.

(b) Meatal projection length

The length of the projection of the earmould into the ear varies the volume of the meatus, which has an effect on the output signal. A long earmould projection will reduce the meatal volume, which will increase the overall sound pressure level and will particularly enhance the low frequency response. A short earmould projection will maintain the volume of the meatus nearer to normal and will therefore provide some enhancement of the higher frequencies.

(c) Venting the earmould

A vent is a hole drilled through the earmould, usually parallel to the sound output channel, although if there is insufficient space in the

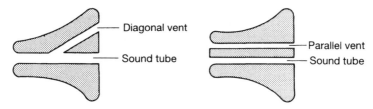

Fig. 9.6 Diagonal and parallel vents. These are used to provide intentional sound leakage, most commonly for the purpose of low frequency reduction.

earmould a diagonal vent opening into the sound tube may be used (Figure 9.6). Venting provides intentional sound leakage and has the greatest effect on the low frequency region. It may be used to relieve a feeling of pressure in the ear or to modify the frequency response of the aid. A small 'pinhole' vent of approximately 0.6 mm will make very little difference to the frequency response but will be effective in allowing pressure equalization, to reduce the feeling of fullness in the ear that many hearing aid users experience.

Many clients have better hearing in the low frequency region and benefit from a reduction of low frequency amplification, which allows them to perceive the important high frequency sounds more clearly. New users also often complain of hearing their voice as hollow or echoing; this is the result of excessive low frequency amplification, generated in the occluded ear and transmitted by bone conduction. It has a noticeable effect on hearing one's own voice and is known as 'the occlusion effect'. Venting is commonly employed for low frequency reduction and is used in conjunction with a short meatal projection for this purpose. It is normal practice to order a vent that is small, medium, large or open ear. The size selected will take into account the gain of the aid and the hearing in the low frequency region, which should be no worse than 30 dBHL if a vent is to be used. In general, the better the hearing in the low frequencies, the larger will be the vent. However, amplified sound leaking from the vent may cause acoustic feedback.

Venting can only be of benefit if the gain of the hearing aid is not sufficient to cause acoustic feedback. An open ear is the largest possible vent size and provides a non-occluding earmould that can only be used if low to moderate gain, over the mid- to high frequency region, is adequate. This type of earmould was originally designed for use with the CROS system and, where it is used on the same ear as the hearing aid, it is sometimes termed an IROS fitting, meaning 'ipsilateral routing of signals' or 'used on the same ear'. An open earmould allows entry of normal unamplified sound, which is useful in many cases of sensorineural hearing loss where the low frequency hearing is good. At the same time, the open ear acts to reduce the amplification of low frequencies below 1.5 kHz, which is obviously not required. However, the open vent does not remove peaks in the frequency response of the aid and its tubing, and the primary peak around 2 kHz can still provide excessive gain for the user unless the peak is damped using an appropriate acoustic filter placed in the tubing or the earhook.

A large vent is usually about 4 mm in diameter and provides strong low frequency reduction below 1 kHz. It is used where the hearing loss below this frequency is not greater than 30 dBHL. If the hearing is good only to 500 Hz, a medium vent with a diameter of 2 mm will reduce the gain adequately. However, the vent itself may resonate causing an increase in gain at a frequency just above the region being reduced, which in some cases may be very undesirable. The problem may be even worse where a small vent is used with the idea of reducing low frequency gain below 250 Hz (Lybarger, 1985). Unless the meatal tip is short and hollowed out the low frequency attenuation is negligible, but there may be a considerable enhancement of perhaps 5 dB to 10 dB at frequencies just above 250 Hz. This is usually not the result that was intended and damping the vent may be necessary to remove the offending peak.

The effect of the vent is sometimes termed 'the vent response'. This is readily found using a probe microphone to measure the difference in sound pressure level in the ear with the earmould vented and with the vent blocked. The vent response interacts with other modifications to provide the required characteristics and it is therefore difficult to establish the precise effect without recourse to real ear measurement. One system that is extremely useful is that often known as the 'select-a-vent' system. The earmould or in-the-ear hearing aid is obtained with a standard-sized hole for which a range of plugs are made. Each plug provides a different-sized vent. The hearing aid audiologist is then able to try various vent sizes without needing to remake the earmould.

(d) Acoustic filters

The frequency response of a hearing aid usually contains two or more peaks of gain. These are due to the effects of the hearing aid electronics and the resonance of the tubing which provides the link between the receiver and the meatus. Peaks of gain may be troublesome because they may cause the output to exceed the user's uncomfortable loudness level, in which case the volume of the aid may be set according to the level of these peaks rather than the overall response of the aid. Acoustic filters, or damping, add a resistance in the sound path, which has the effect of smoothing the resonant peaks. Filters located in the output path have the greatest effect on the midfrequency region between 1 kHz and 3 kHz. The damping effect is maximal when the filter is at the meatal end of the tubing, but this is not very practical because the filter rapidly blocks with wax. For convenience, earhooks are often supplied with damping in place.

The effect of the filters varies not only with their position but also with their acoustic resistance value, which is expressed in ohms. The higher the ohm value, the greater is the smoothing effect. Values from approximately 680 to 4700 ohms are available, but values over about 1500 ohms tend to reduce the midfrequency response to a greater extent than is usually required.

9.3 SUMMARY

Silicone-based materials are recommended for impressions as they undergo little shrinkage. Where a particularly tight acoustic seal is required, addition cured silicone should be used.

An ear examination is important prior to impression-taking and any abnormalities should be noted and, if necessary, referred for medical advice.

Impressions should be taken using the syringe and block method.

Earmoulds can be obtained in a variety of configurations and materials. Hard acrylic is most widely used, since it is an attractive product which is both easy to look after and long-lasting. 'All-soft' materials provide a better acoustic seal but are more difficult to look after and have a much shorter life. Soft acrylic provides a 'half-way house' between hard and all soft materials.

Acoustic modifications can be made to the earmould. These include:

1. Tubing modifications to shift the frequency emphasis. A horn effect can be used to enhance the high frequency response significantly.
2. Alteration to the meatal length. A long meatal length enhances the low frequencies and increases the output. A short meatal length improves the higher frequencies.
3. Venting is commonly used to facilitate limited sound leakage in order to reduce low frequency amplification.
4. Acoustic filters smooth resonant peaks in the frequency response.

The earmould and its plumbing form an integral part of the hearing aid system and can improve or restrict its use.

REFERENCES

Hearing Aid Audiology Group (1994) *The Earmould, Current Practice and Technology*, revised edn (ed. M. Tate), Hearing Aid Audiology Group, British Society of Audiology, Reading.

Lybarger, S. (1985) Earmoulds. *Handbook of Clinical Audiology*, 3rd edn (ed. J.

Katz), Williams and Wilkins, Baltimore, pp. 885–910.
Nolan, M. and Combe, E.C. (1985) Silicone Materials for Ear Impressions. *Scandinavian Audiology*, **14**, 35–9.
Tucker, I. and Nolan, M. (1984) *Educational Audiology*, Croom Helm, London.

FURTHER READING

British Society of Audiology (1986) Recommended Procedure for Taking an Aural Impression. *British Journal of Audiology*, **20**, 315–16.
McHugh, E.R. and Morgan, R. (1988) Earmould/ITE Shell Technology and Acoustics. *Amplification for the Hearing Impaired*, 3rd edn (ed. M. Pollack), Grune and Stratton, Orlando, pp. 105–53.
National Deaf Children's Society (1991) *Recommendations from the Department of Health Seminar on the Production of Earmoulds and Tubing, July 1990*, National Deaf Children's Society, London.

Evaluation   10

10.1 INTRODUCTION

The selection of an appropriate hearing aid and earmould for a client does not signify the end of the hearing aid fitting procedure. Some process must be employed to judge the benefit provided by the aid in terms of its effectiveness and acceptability. Hearing aid evaluation must consider not only the technical dimensions of the aid, but also the subjective opinion of the user, since a hearing aid will provide no benefit unless it is worn.

The prime technical objective is to select and adjust a hearing aid system so that it provides the best possible hearing function. However, this will only be of real benefit if acceptability to the client is not forgotten. There are a number of approaches that can be used to assess:

- the degree to which the aid meets the prescribed characteristics;
- the functional benefits of the hearing aid system;
- the degree to which the aid meets the client's needs and expectations;
- the subjective opinion of the client in relation to sound quality and clarity.

Hearing aid evaluation should be ongoing and viewed as part of an integral approach to audiological rehabilitation.

10.2 INSERTION GAIN MEASUREMENT

Insertion gain provides an objective measure of the gain provided by a hearing aid when worn. Insertion gain procedures involve the placing of a tiny flexible probe tube within the ear canal. The actual sound pressure level is then measured, first without a hearing aid, known as the open ear measurement, and then with the hearing aid in use. The difference between these two measurements is known as the 'insertion gain', and describes the benefit in terms of amplification for the user.

A normal ear acts, in effect, as a natural resonator, amplifying sound entering from the environment or 'sound field'. This amplification is due mainly to ear canal resonance but with some influence from the effects of the pinna and concha (Chapter 2). The gain can vary widely between individuals and even between the left and right ears of the same patient (Tate, 1990). For most patients the gain is usually between 10 dB and 20 dB, but this author has found peak open ear gain to vary from as little as 5 dB to as much as 30 dB in different individuals.

Ear canal resonance is not static throughout life, but changes as the ear grows. In newborn babies the natural resonant peak is near to 6 kHz, but this changes rapidly and the frequency is near that of an adult by about two years of age. The adult peak frequency is between about 2.5 kHz and 3.3 kHz.

When the ear is occluded by an earmould, or an in-the-ear hearing aid, the open ear gain will be altered or lost. This means that when a hearing aid is placed on the ear, that aid has to overcome the loss of natural amplification before it provides any real benefit to the user. Insertion gain corresponds to this benefit.

The terminology surrounding insertion gain (Figure 10.1) can be confusing.

- Insertion gain is the difference between the unaided and aided sound pressure levels measured near the eardrum. The terms

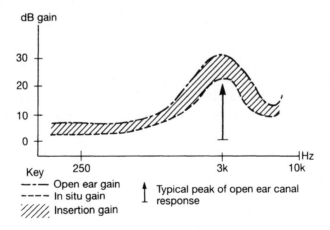

Fig. 10.1 The relationship between *in situ* gain, open ear gain and insertion gain.

etymotic gain, transmission gain and real ear gain are sometimes used to describe insertion gain.
- Open ear gain is the natural amplification afforded by the ear canal resonance and other factors.
- *In situ* measurements are aided measurements taken at the ear without making allowance for the loss of natural amplification.

Insertion gain is the most useful probe tube measurement for hearing aid evaluation. An *in situ* output frequency response could have value in setting the maximum output limit of an aid, but is not generally used in this way.

Prescription methods are often used in the selection of a hearing aid. Real ear gain can be predicted from corrected coupler measurements to provide an approximation that is close to that of the measured real ear gain of an average ear canal. It can be argued that real ear confirmation is not always necessary (Green, 1988), but the disadvantage of the prediction method is that it does not take individual differences into account.

While most patients have an ear canal resonance acceptably close to the average, there are some who differ markedly from it. This will be particularly true at the extremes of age since the ear canals of both young children and the elderly are likely to differ in shape and size from those of the 'average' population. The effect of venting on real ear gain is also very variable, although correction factors appropriate to the vent size will improve the prediction. These problems can be avoided by measuring the real ear gain directly on the client; where a vented mould or shell is used, where the client is very young or very old, or where the results of the fitting appear at variance with the hearing aid audiologist's expectations, real ear insertion gain should be used to clarify the true gain at the ear.

The specialized equipment required for insertion gain measurements can be obtained in a portable form, and for hearing aid fitting purposes may be used in a reasonably quiet, non-sound-treated room. The technique used should, however, be carefully controlled, so that consistent results can be obtained on different test–retest occasions.

As with any method of evaluation there are a number of advantages and disadvantages that should be considered:

Advantages

- Provides an objective measure of real ear performance;
- produces quick and reliable results when used appropriately;
- facilitates accurate modification of the frequency response of the hearing aid;
- can be used with clients unable to perform behavioural tests.

Disadvantages

- Placement of the probe tube requires practice;
- wax deposits in the ear canal may block the probe tube;
- placement of the probe tube may cause unintentional venting leading to an effect on the low frequency response and acoustic feedback;
- does not reduce the importance of more subjective results.

Probe tube measurements can be used to assess how closely a selected hearing aid matches the requirements of gain and output prescribed for the user. If the response is unsatisfactory the effect of modifications, including those to the earmould, can be monitored. Ideally, after the characteristics have been selected and modified according to pre-scription, a more subjective approach should be used to ensure the acceptance of the client is not overlooked. Insertion gain techniques can provide immediate visual feedback for both client and audiologist with regard to the effects of changes made in response to the client's reactions.

10.3 FUNCTIONAL GAIN MEASUREMENT

Functional gain measurements provide another method of assessing the gain provided to the hearing aid user. The method involves the comparison of unaided and aided hearing thresholds, obtained in the 'free-field'.

The difference between the unaided and aided thresholds is termed the 'functional gain'. Functional gain is based on behavioural responses and therefore reflects the efficiency of the auditory system in its entirety.

An audiometer is used to feed warble tones, or narrow bands of noise, through an amplifier to a loudspeaker. This is normally posi-tioned 1 metre in front of the client. The sound pressure level is measured at the client's position using a sound level meter and thresholds are expressed in dBA or dBSPL.

Aided thresholds are sometimes plotted on a pre-printed chart show-ing an average speech spectrum. This will readily indicate the ap-proximate audibility of conversational speech sounds when the aid is worn.

Behavioural thresholds, especially in the free-field, are subject to variability, generally in the order of 5 dB. The difference between unaided and aided thresholds provides an approximate measure of functional gain that correlates reasonably well with insertion gain and which can be usefully compared with prescribed real ear gain.

The acceptability of the selected maximum output of the hearing aid can also be checked by presenting high sound inputs and observing the client's reactions.

Functional gain measurements are most appropriate to use in a sound-treated room and are only widely used in the evaluation of hearing aids for children. Free-field testing of this nature is fairly time-consuming, but can be used to compare the functional gain achieved with prescribed real ear gain, to confirm the adequacy of the aided threshold and to check the client's tolerance at maximum output.

10.4 SPEECH AUDIOMETRY

10.4.1 SPEECH DISCRIMINATION TESTS

Speech discrimination tests are widely used in the evaluation of hearing aid benefit and in clinical diagnosis. The methods used are similar but more rigorously applied for diagnostic purposes. In hearing aid evaluation, the objective is usually:

- to demonstrate the value of a hearing aid;
- to choose the most beneficial aid;
- to demonstrate the value of binaural hearing aids.

Speech audiometry sets out to provide information about the individual's hearing for speech and uses tests given at above threshold intensities. Speech may be delivered to the individual by live voice or recordings.

In the evaluation of a hearing aid system speech tests are undertaken in the free-field, whereas for diagnostic purposes they are usually presented under headphones. Speech audiometry in its broadest sense can provide information concerning hearing for speech, the type and degree of hearing impairment, and the reliability of pure-tone thresholds. Speech tests can provide a useful tool for demonstrating the effectiveness of an appropriately selected hearing aid to the client. Their value in the selection or modification of a hearing aid system is much less reliable.

Speech test scores are very variable and results are not sufficiently precise to correspond to changes in hearing aid performance unless these are extreme. In current practice tests are often used in situations that render them insensitive and unreliable. Where a test is presented using live voice, for example, scores may vary due to uncontrolled changes in voice level. It is therefore important to use 'standardized' test conditions but, even under the most consistent conditions, small variations in speech scores do not indicate significant differences between hearing aid systems. If the limitations are recognized, speech audiometry can serve a useful purpose.

10.4.2 SPEECH TEST MATERIALS

An ideal speech test would:

- be exactly repeatable;
- be phonemically balanced;
- contain words in common usage.

Lists containing words or sentences of equal difficulty are presented. Scores will show some random variation from test to test, but this is minimized by using standardized tests under consistent conditions. Many tests also reflect the same relative balance of phonemes as found in a random sample of everyday speech. This is commonly known as 'phonetic balance' (PB).

Whole lists must be used on each occasion to retain equal difficulty and phonemic or 'phonetic' balance. Whole words are easy to score, but relatively long lists are required to achieve phonetic balance. In the Fry list, for example, Word List 1 consists of:

cut	near	raw	hut	more
sin	keys	tin	ten	thick
bite	lid	sack	less	
will	deaf	men	face	
bone	yard	wish	so	
now	pays	ton	choice	
jam	white	good	veal	
wrong	heard	dip	there	

One entire list must be given at each intensity level in each situation (for instance without and with a hearing aid). This may create a rather long and tiring test. An alternative in widespread use is the presentation of the isophonemic lists of Arthur Boothroyd (1968), commonly known as the AB lists. Each list consists of only ten words, but each word is of consonant-vowel-consonant (CVC) composition. True phonetic balance is not possible within ten words but the same thirty common phonemes are repeated within each list in different combinations (isophonemic).

Each of the separate sounds or phonemes scores one point so, for example, if the test word was 'well', possible verbal responses might be:

Response	Marking	Score
WELL	WELL	3
BELL	WELL	2
WON	WELL	1
TAKE	WELL	0

The nature of the scoring means that guessing should be encouraged, as single correct sounds can appreciably enhance the overall score. A total score of 30 is possible for each list, for example:

AB Word Lists

List 1	List 2	List 3	List 4	List 5
ship	fish	thud	fun	fib
rug	duck	witch	will	thatch
fan	gap	wrap	vat	sum
cheek	cheese	jail	shape	heel
haze	rail	keys	wreath	wide
dice	hive	vice	hide	rake
both	bone	get	guess	goes
well	wedge	shown	comb	shop
jot	moss	hoof	choose	vet
move	tooth	bomb	job	June

In each case the score is presented as a percentage. Monosyllabic word lists are widely used in the UK. Spondees are less frequently used. These are words of two syllables with equal stress on each syllable, for example, 'playground', 'football', 'doorstep'. Spondees are easier to understand but therefore tend to be less sensitive. Maximum scores (100%) are on average achieved at levels 20 dB to 30 dB below those required to achieve maximum scores for monosyllabic words.

Lists of sentences provide a more realistic task than single words. They are somewhat easier and may therefore be less tiring for the listener, but tend to be rather time-consuming. Sentence tests are normally scored by key words. The BKB Sentence Lists (Bench, Kowal and Bamford, 1979) each contain 50 key words, for example:

BKB List 1

The clown had a funny face.

The car engine's running.
She cut with her knife.

Children like strawberries.

The house had nine rooms.

They're buying some bread.

The green tomatoes are small.

He played with his train.

The postman shut the gate.

They're looking at the clock.

The bag bumps on the ground.

The boy did a handstand.

A cat sits on the bed.

The lorry carried fruit.

The rain came down.

The ice cream was pink.

The AB Word Lists and the BKB Lists are used with both older children and adults. Tests for use with younger children must be appropriate to their age and stage of development in terms of the vocabulary presented and the response required.

An oral response is inappropriate for young children who may not have developed sufficient speech skills for the tester to be certain of the response. The Kendall Toy Test is widely used for children in the two-and-a-half to four-year age range. In this test the words in each list are represented by small toys. Fifteen toys are placed on the table in front of the child, ten of which represent test items, the other five are distracters. The child has to point to the appropriate toy when he or she hears the instructions 'Show me the . . .'. The items consist of common vowel and consonant sounds grouped according to the vowel sounds, for example:

Test items: house, spoon, fish, duck, cow, shoe, brick, cup, gate, plate.
Distracters: mouse, book, string, glove, plane.

Picture tests, such as the Manchester Picture Test (Hickson, 1986), are used with slightly older children, from four to six years of age. In this test each word is presented as a multiple choice item. The child is asked 'Show me the . . .' and is required to point to one of four pictures. Each list is designed to test five vowel sounds and five consonant sounds, for example:

Test sound: vowel e.
Pictures presented: well, ball, wall, doll.
Response required: well.

10.4.3 THE SPEECH TEST PROCEDURE

Word lists should be recorded and played through a calibrated system to provide accurate and reliable results. Live voice is prone to great variability in intensity even when it is monitored with a sound level meter, but because of the simplicity of live voice presentation it is widely used for the presentation of word lists in hearing aid evaluation. This should be viewed as informal speech testing; the term 'speech audiometry' should be reserved for tests presented under measurable and reproducible conditions. Speech audiometry generally makes use of an audiometer to pass the signal to the patient through headphones or via an amplifier and loudspeaker. Part 2 of IEC 645 (equivalent to BS 5966) specifies the requirements for speech audiometers.

An audiometer for speech tests will have the facility to accept the signal from a microphone or tape recorder and should also be able to provide masking for speech using white noise or speech spectrum noise, which contains more low frequency noise. IEC 645 and BS 5966 (1980) provide for speech spectrum noise to fall by 12 dB per octave between 1 kHz and 6 kHz. Masking with both kinds of noise is equally effective, but speech spectrum noise is less fatiguing since it excludes unnecessary high frequency energy. Masking will be required in speech audiometry, if results are required for each ear separately, where the pure-tone audiogram suggests that cross-hearing may occur.

Pre-recorded speech tests are prefaced with a 20 dBSPL, 1 kHz calibration tone of at least 1 minute in length; this is used to check that the input level to the audiometer is the same every time it is used and that the dial settings are therefore consistent. The calibration tone should measure 20 dBSPL when the hearing level control on the audiometer is set to zero, or the level indicator is set to its reference point.

Speech audiometry should be carried out in quiet conditions to minimize the masking effects of background noise. This is particularly important for free-field tests. The background noise should be measured and should not be such as to interfere with a signal to noise ratio of 45 dB.

A standard speech audiogram cannot be produced because differences in test materials and conditions may affect results. Each speech set-up must therefore provide its own normal response curve to which patients' responses will be compared. This can be achieved by testing a group, usually of 20, normally-hearing adults under exactly the same test conditions as are to be used with all patients. A number of word lists must be given at different presentation levels and the results at each presentation level are averaged to produce a normal response curve.

Patients should be given careful instructions. These should include that they will hear someone speaking single words (or sentences) and after each word they should repeat any parts of the word they heard.

10.4.4 SPEECH TESTS FOR DIAGNOSTIC PURPOSES

The first word list should be presented at a comfortable level and used for practice and to adjust the starting point if the patient is not scoring well. The intensity level is increased or decreased in 10 dB or 20 dB

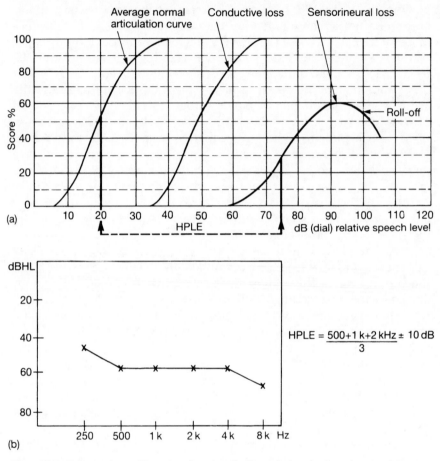

Fig. 10.2 A speech audiogram showing half-peak level elevation and its relation to the pure-tone audiogram.

steps, with one full list given at each level, and the scores are plotted on a speech audiogram.

Where monosyllabic word lists are used in speech audiometry, half peak level (HPL) is proposed as a measure that agrees well with the pure-tone audiogram. HPL is the intensity (in dial units) at which the patient obtains half of his or her maximum score, whatever that maximum may be. Thus, if a patient has a maximum score of 100, the HPL will be 50, but if the maximum score is only 60, the HPL will be 30. The difference between the normal HPL and the patient's HPL is known as the 'half peak level elevation' (HPLE) (Figure 10.2).

The HPLE elevation should agree, within 10 dB, with the pure-tone audiogram averaged over 500 Hz, 1 kHz and 2 kHz. Where the HPLE does not agree, a greater shift may indicate an inaccurate audiogram, or, rarely, point towards a retrocochlear disorder. Where the shift is less than predicted, this is likely to indicate a non-organic disorder.

• The shape of the speech curve for a typical conductive loss will follow the shape of the normal reference curve, but will be displaced or shifted along the audiogram. The patient will reach a score of 100% but at an intensity level that is elevated in comparison with the normal.

In the case of a typical sensorineural loss the discrimination curve is again shifted but may never reach a 100% score. The patient achieves his or her maximum score at some lower percentage score and when the intensity is increased beyond this point, the score reduces, shown by a 'roll over' on the audiogram.

Speech audiometry is a useful tool in the assessment of how an individual's hearing for speech varies with intensity, both with and without a hearing aid.

A simplified procedure may be used to provide a simple comparison of hearing aid benefit, where the recorded material is delivered at a constant sound level, usually 60 dB or 70 dB, 1 metre from the loud-speaker. At least one word list is presented at this level for each of the aids, or situations, to be compared. A comparison of unaided and aided discrimination scores is likely to show an improvement (except with a very mild hearing loss) even with a poorly selected hearing aid. Nevertheless, the comparison can be useful to demonstrate to a new client that it will be beneficial to wear a hearing aid.

10.5 SUBJECTIVE EVALUATION

A hearing aid system will only be of benefit if it is worn. Client acceptability must therefore be taken into account in any evaluation. A number of methods of obtaining the client's subjective opinion exists, with regard to both the sound quality of the aid and its functional benefit.

In many cases, the information is obtained through interview or discussion with the client, informally structured to:

• provide information regarding the sound quality;
• provide information about the usefulness of the aid;
• identify situations that remain problematic.

The information obtained may lead to adjustment of the system or to further rehabilitation. Questions regarding sound quality can be tailored to provide information that will indicate the need for certain modifications, for example:

Is the aid loud enough?   – adjustment of gain
Is the aid clear enough?   – adjustment of bass cut (high-pass filter)
Is the sound tinny or harsh? – adjustment of treble cut (low-pass filter)

Quality judgements are not particularly useful for choosing between hearing aids as there is a marked tendency for clients to select the second of two aids, that is to select merely by order rather than due to any particular attributes of the aid itself (Green, Day and Bamford, 1989).

Quality judgements are useful in achieving hearing aid satisfaction and can be helpful in making decisions with regard to aid modifications. In some cases, a measurement scale may be used. The client is asked to listen to a passage of running speech and to judge sound quality between two examples, on a scale of one to five, for instance. This is completed for a number of paired attributes, such as loud/soft, clear/hazy, booming/shrill, pleasant/unpleasant. Alternatively, the client may be asked questions tailored to indicate the need for modifications.

There is a tendency for clients to dislike high frequency emphasis at first fitting, even when this can be shown to improve their speech discrimination. With long-term experience of using hearing aids, many clients will come to accept a higher emphasis frequency response. Evaluation after an extended period of rehabilitation will allow maximum advantage to be taken of the client's gradual acclimatization to hearing aid use.

A questionnaire may also form part of an evaluation after a period of rehabilitation, and should be designed to indicate particular problem areas, as well as the overall level of satisfaction. A disability questionnaire can be given before, and some time after, hearing aid fitting to indicate the difficulties the client originally had and to what extent the aid has reduced the client's problems. Questions are presented in a way that allows improvements to be readily noted, for example:

> Can you follow the television news when the volume is turned up only enough to suit other people?
> Easily
> With some difficulty
> With great difficulty
> Not at all
>
> *Lutman, Brown and Coles, 1987*

If a simple individual questionnaire, or even a checklist, is to be designed to identify particular difficulties it may be useful to indicate:

- how long the aid is worn each day;
- the ease of insertion, manipulation and removal;
- comfort;
- feedback problems;
- satisfaction with the appearance;

- perceived sound quality;
- difficulties encountered in (a) the home; (b) at work; (c) socially;
- satisfaction with the hearing aid;
- satisfaction with the service.

10.6 SUMMARY

Evaluation is an important part of the overall process of hearing aid fitting. Methods in common use include:

- insertion gain;
- functional gain;
- speech audiometry;
- subjective evaluation.

Methods of evaluation should be chosen to provide information about benefit in terms of:

- adequacy of prescribed characteristics;
- comfort;
- reduction of handicap;
- sound quality.

The results should highlight any problem areas and lead to modifications and further rehabilitation where appropriate.

REFERENCES

Bench, J., Kowal, A. and Bamford, J.M. (1979) The BKB (Bamford-Kowal-Bench) Sentence Lists for Partially Hearing Children. *British Journal of Audiology*, **13**, 108–12.

Boothroyd, A. (1968) *The Arthur Boothroyd (AB) Word Lists*, Manchester University, Manchester.

British Standards Institution (1980) *BS 5966: Specification for Audiometers*, British Standards Institution, London.

Green, R. (1988) The Relative Accuracy of Coupler and Behavioural Estimates of the Real Ear Gain of a Hearing Aid. *British Journal of Audiology*, **22**, 35–44.

Green, R., Day, S. and Bamford, J. (1989) A Comparative Evaluation of Four Hearing Aid Selection Procedures, II – Quality Judgements as Measures of Benefit. *British Journal of Audiology*, **23**, 201–6.

Hickson, F. (1986) *The Manchester Picture Test*, Manchester University.

Lutman, M.E., Brown, E.J. and Coles, R.R.A. (1987) Self-Reported Disability and Handicap in the Population in Relation to Pure-Tone Threshold, Age, Sex and Type of Hearing Loss. *British Journal of Audiology*, **21**(1), 45–58.

Tate, M. (1990) The Application of Real Ear Probe Tube Measurements to Hearing Aid Fitting. *Acoustic Letters*, **14**(1), 1–6.

FURTHER READING

Pollack, M.C. (1988) *Amplification for the Hearing-Impaired*, 3rd edn, Grune and Stratton, Orlando.
Tucker, I. and Nolan, M. (1984) *Educational Audiology*, Croom Helm, Beckenham.

Client management and rehabilitation 11

11.1 THE REHABILITATION PROCESS

The most common cause of acquired hearing loss in adulthood is the result of the ageing process (presbyacusis). About 8% of the adult population have a hearing loss over 35 dB in the better ear (Haggard, Gatehouse and Davies, 1981), while approximately one-third of the population over 65 years old has some sort of hearing problem, and approximately half of the population over 80 years old has a severe hearing problem. Hearing losses of this type develop gradually over a period of years, with high frequency sounds reducing first. This means that speech can still be heard, but it loses its clarity. A binaural hearing loss of as little as 15 dBHL, averaged across the frequencies 500 Hz to 2 kHz, is likely to be significantly disabling for everyday speech (Lutman, Brown and Coles, 1987). An affected individual typically accuses others of mumbling or speaking quietly, and this leads to increased tensions within the family. Although hearing loss may be suspected, this is not usually a suggestion that is readily accepted by the hearing impaired person, who often prefers to cope with the restriction of personal and social life rather than admit to deafness. In many cases there may be a gap of as much as 15 years or more between noticing the problem and taking any action to deal with it.

Hearing loss is an underestimated impairment that may lead to many secondary problems in addition to primary communication difficulties. Management of the hearing impaired client is extremely difficult and, unless the client accepts the problem, rejection of any form of hearing aid is very likely. Even when the need for amplification is understood, deafness remains an unacceptable condition and most people would prefer to use an inconspicuous hearing aid. Indeed, although commercial aids provide a wide choice of size, type and frequency response, most of those people who choose to use private hearing aids do so for cosmetic reasons (Rendell *et al.*, 1992).

High expectations of the benefit to be derived from hearing aids add to the difficulties, especially as most adults do not realize hearing loss is not 'cured' by amplification. Hearing aids alone are not sufficient to overcome the consequences of the loss. Audiological rehabilitation involving a co-ordinated programme of evaluation and remedy is therefore appropriate.

Aural rehabilitation begins with an evaluation of the hearing loss and its effect on the client's life-style. At this stage it is decided if remediation is necessary and, if it is, whether hearing aids should be considered. In some cases assistive devices may be sufficient to ful-fil the client's needs. If hearing aids are to be considered, and fol-lowing referral to a medical practitioner if indicated (section 6.1.1), the acoustical characteristics can be defined, together with any special rehabilitation measures required. It is usually helpful to include a member or members of the client's family in the process, as not only can they support the hearing impaired person far better if they under-stand, but also concerns are more likely to be aired at an early stage. Rehabilitation is not really an area on its own but is interwoven into hearing aid fitting and evaluation. The success of the whole process is reliant on the sum of the individual parts. An error in any part may adversely affect the whole, for example, incorrect uncomfortable loud-ness levels (ULLs) could lead to the fitting of a hearing aid that is too loud. The aid might appear suitable in the quiet of the fitting situation, but in the noise of the outside world prove unbearable. The client could turn it down but then would not hear adequately, leading to rejection of the aid. Another example could be where the hearing aid audiologist fails to consider the patient's dexterity, leading to the selec-tion of an aid that the client is unable to insert or operate.

The aid type suggested must be acceptable to the client such that he or she is both able and willing to wear it and, if it is a commercial aid, it must be affordable. These and many other factors interact in the audiological rehabilitation process. The client's attitude towards hearing impairment and amplification is crucial to the rehabilitative process, and four attitude types have been outlined (Goldstein and Stevens, 1981):

Type I – the patient has a very positive attitude towards hearing aids and aural rehabilitation.

Type II – is an essentially positive attitude but with some complicating factors present. These might, for example, include a pre-viously unfavourable hearing aid fitting experience, or a difficult-to-fit hearing loss.

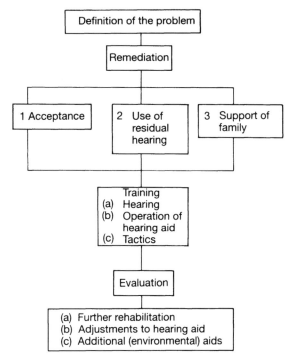

Fig. 11.1 A problem-solving model of the rehabilitation process.

Type III – is an essentially negative attitude but with an element of co-operative intent.

Type IV – consists of a small group who reject hearing aids completely. Unfortunately, rehabilitation is rarely successful with this group.

A simple problem-solving model of the rehabilitation process is presented in Figure 11.1. The process begins with a definition of the problem. At this stage the hearing aid audiologist collects information regarding the client's hearing loss, his or her areas of difficulty, his or her attitude and related aspects. Informal discussion, a case history and audiological assessment are the most widely used tools for defining the problem. Handicap questionnaires and speech audiometry may add further depth to the investigations.

The focus of any rehabilitation process should be on the needs of the individual, and aural rehabilitation can be defined as helping an individual with a specific set of problems arising from an auditory disorder. Rehabilitation can therefore be considered as a process that is designed to minimize disability due to hearing loss or tinnitus (and to some extent, balance) in order to prevent the condition from handicapping the client.

The hearing problem can be viewed as a continuum in which disability and handicap represent different stages. Initially, damage to the auditory system leads to impairment or hearing loss. This creates a disability, but it is the degree to which this disability affects a person's quality of life and well-being that imposes the handicap.

Thus, for example, a moderate hearing loss might have only a slight handicapping effect on an elderly client living alone, seeing few visitors and whose only real problem seems to be hearing the television. An identical degree of hearing loss in a young married man could cause a considerable handicap. The disability of the hearing impairment is likely to affect every aspect of his life-style and employment because of its impact on communication. Activities that were previously enjoyable become difficult and he is likely to experience embarrassment, irritation, frustration, anger and depression. He will almost certainly perceive a change in his status, at least in his own eyes, and will suffer a loss of self-esteem.

The need to wear a hearing aid is generally regarded as related to the ageing process and society makes few allowances for hearing impairment. Unlike wearing spectacles, where the individual may be considered intelligent and studious, hearing aids carry a stigma. They are an external sign of deafness, which many view as being accompanied by stupidity because of the communication problem it creates. Spectacles may result in perfect vision. A hearing aid rarely produces an immediate return to normal, but is much in parallel with the use of a wheelchair. Socially, hearing loss produces less sympathy and understanding than the loss of a limb.

Hearing loss is rarely total, and the person who hears some things and not others is described as awkward, 'he hears when he wants to'. In background noise and group situations, following a conversation may be impossible. The hearing impaired person wants to maintain social interaction but restricted involvement in conversations has to be tolerated. Some attempt may be made at finding a way of controlling the social scene or avoiding it (Hallberg and Carlsson, 1991). Often, particularly in the early stages, the hearing impaired person will prefer to isolate himself socially.

The objectives of the first stage in the rehabilitation process, then, are to assess the impairment through audiometry, and the nature of the handicap through investigation of the client's home, work and social environment, the activities in which he or she wishes or needs to participate and the difficulties being experienced. Only when the problem has been defined can a realistic approach to remediation be adopted.

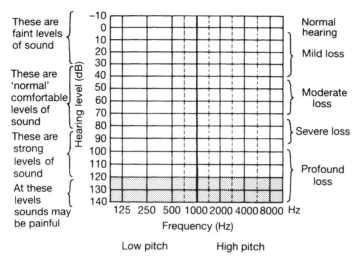

Fig. 11.2 Audiometric information that can be readily explained to the client.

The remediation process involves more than just hearing aid fitting. It involves setting the scene to facilitate the best possible use of amplification. There are some individuals for whom hearing aids may not be appropriate, and sometimes assistive devices, such as a television amplifier, may provide a successful answer to a specific need. Where hearing aids are appropriate, counselling is often required to help the person come to terms with his or her loss and accept realistically the impairment and ensuing handicap. If the client maintains a type III attitude, with perhaps only a grudging acceptance of a problem, much counselling may be needed to achieve acceptance. Even where clients maintain positive, type I, attitudes, counselling is equally required to help them understand the potential benefits and limitations of amplification. The client needs to understand that hearing aids will not provide perfect hearing and, while they can be of great benefit, it will take time to relearn to associate sounds with meanings. A positive attitude is undoubtedly helpful but unrealistic expectations will lead to disappointment and the possible rejection of any amplification system. Most adults are interested to know about their hearing loss and to understand the difficulties they experience. At an early stage the type and degree of loss and the audiogram can be explained (Figure 11.2). Understanding may help to increase acceptance.

If the hearing loss is of sudden onset the impact is much greater than a loss that has developed slowly and insidiously over many years. The patient has not had time to compensate for the loss or to come to terms with it. The hearing impaired person (or the parents of the hearing impaired child) need time and empathetic counselling to move through stages of grief and mourning at their loss before they are ready to understand or accept. Such stages can be identified as follows.

Stage I – numbness

It is usually the ENT surgeon or otolaryngologist that is involved at this point to provide direct advice on handling the impairment. Unfortunately, the client is often unable to absorb much of the information given at this stage.

Stage II – denial

The client refuses to accept the diagnosis and searches for a second opinion or a miracle cure. The client is not yet ready for amplification and if hearing aids are prescribed they are unlikely to be used. 'Initial strategies involve denying disability, pretending to hear and avoidance of situations in which the disability will be exposed. The deafened person looks to medicine for a cure to problems which are seen as stemming from faults in the ear. When the cure is not forthcoming, the deafened person experiences a further loss – that of hope.' (Woolley, 1991).

Stage III – despair

This is the stage at which the hearing loss is accepted but the problems often appear insurmountable. Positive but realistic counselling of the client and his or her family can help the client to move towards acceptance of the problems and a desire to try to overcome them.

Stage IV – action

The client is ready to accept amplification. Counselling and training now interlink to facilitate the client's adjustment to the impairment and to the use of amplification.

Whatever the degree of loss and the pattern of its onset, involvement of the family or a 'significant other' is important as their help and support can be of immense value. A 'significant other' is anyone who is in close and frequent contact with the client and will often be the spouse or a son or daughter. Their presence throughout the rehabilitation process, at the assessment, hearing aid fitting and aftercare, can help them to understand the nature of the problem. Their expectations also have to be realistic and they need to realize that it takes time and effort to overcome the handicap of deafness. They also are affected by the loss and they need to understand the problems of poor speech discrimination, difficulty in noise, recruitment and so on if they are to be able to provide realistic support and encouragement to the hearing impaired person. They can also ensure that practical instructions have been understood and, if necessary, can help in inserting the aid and in its care.

11.2 PRACTICAL ASPECTS OF REHABILITATION

11.2.1 PRACTICAL INSTRUCTION

First-time hearing aid users will require training in effective hearing aid use, which can be considered as 'informational counselling'. Such counselling is also required to a lesser extent when a client changes from one hearing aid system to another, or from monaural use to binaural.

11.2.2 INSERTION AND REMOVAL OF THE AID

Difficulty in inserting the earmould or hearing aid is the most common reason for lack of use. It is an activity that has to be learned through practice, and it is essential to ensure that the client or his or her carer is able to insert and remove the aid at the hearing aid fitting stage, while the hearing aid audiologist is on hand to provide guidance. It is a common fault for clients to leave the top part of the helix of the earmould outside the fold of the pinna. It may be helpful for the 'significant other' to be shown how the aid should appear when properly inserted (Figure 11.3).

Where there is some difficulty in manual ability half shell moulds may provide a useful option as these are easier to insert and a small handle can be fitted to help in removal. Very small hearing aids with very small controls and tiny batteries are only appropriate if the client can handle them satisfactorily – no matter how good the amplification or how much the client wants a small aid.

11.2.3 OPERATING THE AID

New users need precise simple instruction on operating and care of the hearing aid. They must be sure of the size and type of battery to use. If they are using zinc air batteries they need to be aware that removal of the tab will cause the battery to deteriorate. It is common for a user to try several new batteries, one after the other, if the hearing aid does not work. The use of a battery cell tester to ensure the adequacy of the battery current can avoid this problem since the client can then be

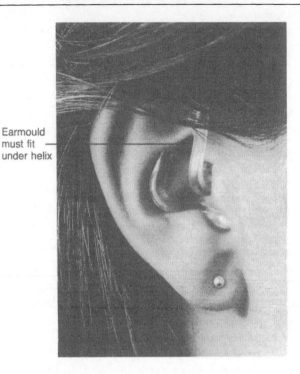

Earmould
must fit
under helix

Fig. 11.3 The appearance of an earmould when correctly inserted. (Photograph courtesy of P.C. Werth Ltd.)

certain whether it is the battery at fault. Insertion of the battery can be difficult with poor eyesight or failing dexterity. It is sensible to change batteries over a towel (on the table or on the knees) as it is much easier to retrieve a small battery in this way. The client needs to realize that the battery has a positive flat side, and a negative rounded side. The battery must be in the drawer the correct way around, with the positive side matching the positive sign shown on the aid. If it is placed back to front the battery drawer will not close easily, and it should never be forced shut. Clients also need information about how to dispose of old batteries safely, where to obtain new supplies and how often they will need to replace them. The aid should be turned off when not in use to reduce battery consumption and it is sometimes helpful to suggest that the battery compartment be opened at night to ensure there is no unnecessary drain. Most clients will want to know how long a battery should last, and a reasonable indication of battery life should be possible, taking account of the hearing aid manufacturer's information and the client's probable usage. Further information on calculating battery life will be found in section 7.6.2. When the battery has run out, it should never be thrown in the fire or left where pets or children may swallow it. Swallowed batteries are extremely dangerous: ingestion of any battery is potentially lethal and medical attention should be obtained without delay.

New users may be concerned about the volume at which to set their new aids, and without advice often set them too high or too low. They need to understand that the volume should be adjusted in different situations but, as a starting point, it is often helpful to encourage the client to rotate the volume control until the aid is a little too loud and then reduce it slightly. Alternatively, the aid may be pre-set using a test box or insertion gain. A prescription formula or the subtraction of an average conversational level (60 dB to 70 dB) from the most comfortable level may provide the basis for this approach. However, even when the gain is pre-set, the client should not normally use this setting in all situations. A spot of nail varnish to mark the appropriate volume setting can be helpful where a parent or carer sets the aid. Children should be encouraged to take responsibility for their own aids, including setting the volume, as early as possible. Many children of five years old are able to approach this sensibly, although parents and teachers need to keep an eye on the situation!

Binaural hearing aids can be adjusted in the same manner as monaural aids, but both aids will then need to be turned down slightly and adjusted as necessary to ensure that sound is heard centrally. If the loss is very asymmetrical or the client has become used to listening monaurally over a long period of time, it may be better not to attempt to 'balance' the ears in this way, at least initially.

If the hearing aid includes other client-operated controls, such as telecoil, tone controls or an on–off switch, these must be demonstrated and their use practised at the initial fitting stage. A common problem is where a client switches to the 'T' position for receiving from a loop, but forgets to return the aid to the normal 'M' position afterwards and therefore thinks the aid is faulty. Practice in use can be arranged at the fitting stage by attaching a telecoil adaptive coupler to the telephone, and using the speaking clock or similar service.

Induction loops are frequently installed in churches and other public places but most modern domestic telephones do not have the telecoil facility, hence the need for a special adaptive coupler to provide practice at the early stages.

A further aspect of hearing aid operation the client should understand is when and why feedback may occur. A correctly-fitted hearing aid should not feedback in normal usage, but it is likely if the aid is not inserted correctly, if the microphone is covered with a hat or hand, or if the ear is blocked with wax. Clients can be helped to understand feedback by explaining that it occurs when amplified sound escapes from the ear canal and re-enters the microphone of the hearing aid such that it is re-amplified and heard as a high-pitched whistle. If the aid has to be turned down below the required volume to prevent feedback, the hearing aid audiologist must find and rectify the cause, perhaps by reducing the vent size or making a new tighter-fitting earpiece.

Feedback can be used to advantage in checking the battery. If the aid is held in a cupped hand, with the volume fully on, and the aid does not whistle the battery can usually be assumed to be dead.

11.2.4 CARE OF THE AID

Hearing aids are small, expensive items and new users need to be informed how to care for their aids. They may not realize that the aid should not come into contact with water, make-up, hair spray and perfume. Batteries should be removed if aids are not used for a long period and aids should be kept away from extreme temperatures. An earmould can be separated from the hearing aid and washed in warm water, although care should be taken to ensure no moisture remains in the tubing before reconnection to the aid. An air blower or 'puffer' can be used to remove moisture (including condensation after use) from the tubing. In-the-ear hearing aids must not be washed. Cleaning involves wiping them periodically with a dry tissue or cloth and checking the sound outlet and vent, if applicable, for wax when the aid is removed each night. Wax can be removed carefully using a special wax tool or small cleaning brush, with the receiver outlet over a tissue to collect the debris as it falls out. Nothing should be inserted down the sound outlet further than about 5 mm as damage to the receiver could result. A small metal or plastic wax trap may be fitted by the manufacturer to prevent any wax particles finding their way into the receiver. This does not reduce the need for the client to clean the opening, but if the trap becomes blocked the hearing aid audiologist will usually need to clean it for the client. Cream or Vaseline, which some clients use to ease insertion of the aid, can also block and damage the aid unless used sparingly and with care. Dirt in the receiver and in the microphone are common causes of hearing aid damage. The aid should therefore be handled with clean, dry hands and should be removed during potentially damaging situations, such as washing or shaving.

For many first-time users there seems to be a great deal of information to assimilate, and written instructions for operation and care should also be provided. Clients should be encouraged to read these in the first few days.

11.2.5 TRAINING IN HEARING AND FIRST USE OF THE AID

Most new users need to become acclimatized to hearing aid use over a period of time. They are usually advised to build up their use gradually from an hour or two in quiet surroundings. At first they are usually advised not to try to 'test' the aid, but to restrict use to reasonably easy situations, such as conversation with single members of the family, or listening to news programmes on the television. The news is helpful because the newsreader faces the audience and provides clear speech, without background noise or a complex story line to follow. It is usually inadvisable for the aids to be worn too soon in noisy situations, and it is therefore not sensible for the client to wear the hearing aid in the street immediately after fitting. Wind and traffic noise are particularly disconcerting. The approach should, however, be flexible and individual: not every client needs to build up use, and this is often particularly true of younger clients. A client should not be prevented from wearing the aid for as long as he or she likes, provided that it is turned down if the sound is too loud or taken off if the aid is uncomfortable or the client becomes tired.

In the early stages of hearing aid use, or of change to a different system, the client may be unable to tolerate the prescribed pattern of amplification. A seemingly appropriate high-frequency emphasis may appear to sound 'tinny' or the aid may seem too loud. It may be necessary to provide a high frequency cut, or to reduce the output through peak clipping, or perhaps to provide some AGC. When the client becomes acclimatized to hearing aid use their tolerance will often increase, and it is usually possible with tone controls or programmable aids to alter the aid's controls gradually to maximize the client's benefit from the amplification system.

After-care is an important part of the rehabilitation process. The client must be able to contact the hearing aid audiologist if problems or queries arise. A few clients do not need further help, but most appreciate subsequent information and attention, which may ease acceptance of the aid. Evaluation, whether formal or informal, should be built into the rehabilitation programme and lead on to adjustments to the hearing aids, further rehabilitation and perhaps the addition of other 'assistive' devices to help overcome specific problems. When the rehabilitation period is satisfactorily completed, contact with the client is usually maintained through servicing tasks, such as retubing or cleaning battery contacts, and providing regular hearing checks. Often the client will be interested in new products and the hearing aid audiologist should be ready to provide factual information about assistive devices and new types of hearing aids.

11.2.6 TACTICS

Many of the difficulties caused by hearing loss can be minimized by the use of some simple hearing 'tactics'. Over time, the hearing impaired person may develop his or her own set of tactics, but the hearing aid audiologist may help ease the early stages with a few practical suggestions, which might include the following:

1. Reduce background noise – turn off the radio or other competing noise, hold a conversation in the lounge rather than the hall, use a tablecloth to reduce the clatter of plates, and so on. The hearing aid volume may also be turned down a little in noisy situations.
2. Ensure adequate lighting – the room should be well lit and the lights should fall on the speaker's face not in the client's eyes.
3. Positioning – reduction of the distance between listener and speaker will improve hearing; a distance of about 1 metre is ideal for lip-reading and is not uncomfortably close.
4. Encouraging others – it is helpful if the attention of the hearing impaired person is attracted, perhaps by calling a name and then pausing, before a conversation is started. The speaker should be encouraged to face the client and speak clearly, to make the subject of the conversation known and to rephrase anything not fully understood. Shouting and speaking very slowly with exaggerated lip movements do not help, but slowing speech slightly, using clear speech and a loud voice will help. Good communication demands an effort from both the listener and the speaker.

Even people with a very mild hearing loss can benefit from the introduction of hearing tactics. With a more severe loss, there may be an increased reliance not only on tactics but also on speech-reading.

11.2.7 LIP-READING AND AUDITORY TRAINING

Lip-reading can be a useful adjunct to a hearing aid user with any degree of impairment. Even with normal hearing we use lip-reading to some extent in difficult listening situations. Some individuals acquire great skill in lip-reading without conscious effort but, for most, lip-reading is a difficult task.

I tried to lip-read. I had not expected to understand much but the reality was a choking experience. I understood very little of what was said and, to add to my discomfort, I had no idea where to look. By the time I swivelled round to locate a speaker he would be half-way through his question; a brief one would be finished before I could start to make any sense of it . . . As shadows flitted across the faces I was trying to lip-read they made a difficult task impossible.

Ashley, 1991

Lip-reading classes are often provided through the local education authority, where the hearing impaired can obtain help in developing the skill. Although it would appear that lip-reading is 'caught' rather than taught, classes can provide graded practice and encouragement. In addition, bringing people with similar problems together provides a degree of group therapy, which may be very helpful in developing understanding, acceptance and a more positive and assertive attitude.

Individuals who have a more severe or profound hearing loss of long-standing may benefit from auditory training. This is a series of exercises designed to help the deaf person to learn to listen and to build up the correct associations of sounds and their meanings. Sessions are usually individual and may be provided by hearing therapists, speech and language therapists or teachers of the deaf. Sign language and finger-spelling are rarely used by adults with acquired deafness because they are of little help in communicating with the hearing community.

11.3 ASSISTIVE DEVICES FOR THE HEARING IMPAIRED

11.3.1 AUXILIARY AIDS

There are many devices to help the hearing impaired either in addition to, or in place of, hearing aids. Such devices are known as 'environmental aids', 'assistive devices' or 'auxiliary aids', and they are designed to assist with specific everyday problems, such as listening to the television, or on the telephone. Many of these use an induction loop or an infra-red system, and for the more severely deaf visual or vibrating indicators are often used, particularly for alarm sounds and for the doorbell and telephone. Details of current assistive devices can be obtained from the RNID (Royal National Institute for Deaf People) or from the various manufacturers. Many of the special systems available may be obtained on free loan through the local social services department, although availability depends on local finances and policies; alternatively clients may purchase devices privately. Where special systems are required to aid someone in employment, it may be possible to obtain these through the local Job Centre.

11.3.2 THE INDUCTION LOOP SYSTEM

An induction loop system is designed to enable a sound signal to be transmitted directly to the listener. This overcomes problems created by background noise, reverberation and increasing distance from the sound source. The loop utilizes the principle of electromagnetic induction.

(a) Electromagnetic induction

A current flowing in a wire creates a magnetic field around it. The loop system involves a cable fitted around the required area and attached to an amplifier. The sound source is fed into the amplifier through a microphone, or by a direct connection from the television or other device.

When a suitable pick-up receiver enters the magnetic field, the sound signals are transmitted to it by a fluctuating magnetic signal from the loop cable. Most behind-the-ear, and some in-the-ear hearing aids are fitted with this facility, which is known as the 'T' switch. (Modern telephones do not produce an adequate magnetic field for the operation of the induction loop, unless this is specifically designed for.) When the wearer switches to 'T', only signals from the loop system may be heard. If the wearer also wishes to hear sounds from the environment, to hear friends talking for instance, the aid must be fitted with a switch that allows the microphone to remain operative; this is known as an 'MT' switch. Where a hearing aid is not in use, separate induction loop receivers can be supplied.

(b) Loop design

The installation of a domestic loop system is a relatively simple matter. For a loop system to operate successfully in a public place and to meet all the necessary requirements (British Standards Institution, 1981), specialized design and installation are essential.

The major disadvantages of the loop system are:

1. Overspill interference will result where two loop systems are used in adjacent rooms.
2. The frequency response on 'T' may be different to the normal reception on 'M'. In particular the low frequency response may be less good.
3. Weak or dead spots can arise within the looped area.
4. There may be electrical interference that generates internal noise in the hearing aid, near fluorescent lights, for example.
5. Orientation of the head may cause variation in the gain received of as much as 15 dB (Tucker and Nolan, 1984).

11.4 MANAGEMENT PRACTICES

11.4.1 THE ROLE OF THE HEARING AID AUDIOLOGIST

Hearing aid audiologists usually undertake the total aural rehabilitation of clients who have chosen to obtain a hearing aid through a private route. Their primary responsibility is therefore to ensure that hearing impaired clients obtain maximum benefit from their hearing aid system. In order to achieve this, they will determine:

- the need for medical referral;
- the hearing loss;
- the client's difficulties and feelings in relation to the hearing problem;
- the need for a hearing aid.

The hearing aid audiologist should guide and support clients in their search for solutions to their hearing problems. This will usually, but not always, involve the selection and adjustment of a hearing aid system together with the provision of rehabilitation counselling and after-care service to ensure that the system provides maximum benefit to the client.

11.4.2 THE HEARING AID COUNCIL CODE OF PRACTICE

The Hearing Aid Council Act of 1968 provides for 'the establishment of a Hearing Aid Council, to register persons engaged in the supply of hearing aids, to advise on the training of persons engaged in such business, and to regulate trade practices'. The Hearing Aid Council (Amendment) Act of 1989 introduced changes to the composition of the council and extended its disciplinary powers. On a day-to-day basis the Hearing Aid Council (HAC) is administered by a Registrar, but the council itself consists of 12 members, four to represent the interests of the hearing impaired consumer, four with specialized medical or audiological technical knowledge and four to represent the interests of the private hearing aid dispenser. The council members are appointed by the Department of Trade and Industry (DTI) and each serves a three-year term, although this may be followed by one further term of three years. The full council meets four times a year, and there are additional meetings of its standing committees – the Examining Committee, Complaints Investigating Committee and Disciplinary Committee.

The main functions of the Hearing Aid Council are the establishment and maintenance of standards of competence and the regulation of trade practices. These are achieved through implementation of the HAC's Code of Practice and the complaints and disciplinary procedures. Included in the Code of Practice (1990) are 29 numbered clauses that regulate all aspects of dispensing practice. The following provides a summary of the main provisions in relation to dispensers.

(a) Self-representation

Hearing aid dispensers may not use misleading or unqualified descriptions such as 'consultant', 'specialist' or 'audiologist' unless preceded by the words 'hearing aid', nor may they designate their premises as a clinic or institute, and specified wording, relating to registration under the Act, must be used.

(b) Medical referral

Dispensers must advise clients to seek medical advice (if they have not already done so) if they complain of or show any of the following:

- excessive wax in the ear;
- discharge from the ear;
- vertigo;
- earache;
- deafness of short duration or of sudden onset;
- unilateral sensorineural hearing loss;
- conductive hearing loss;
- tinnitus;
- exposure to loud noise at work or elsewhere.

(c) Facilities

Premises must provide a suitable reception or waiting room, a self-contained private examination room, a suitable storage system for confidential client records and a room for audiometry that is not subject to excessive noise. At every consultation, there must be available:

- a regularly calibrated pure-tone audiometer with facilities for air and bone conduction with masking;
- an otoscope and specula, with facilities for cleaning them;
- aural impression material and equipment;
- a range of air and bone conduction hearing aids.

It must also be possible to arrange speech audiometry when required. Appropriate air and bone conduction audiometry must be carried out unless the dispenser has available an audiogram taken within the previous two months by or under supervision of an ENT surgeon.

(d) Information for clients

At all times dispensers should provide the best possible advice including, where appropriate, that a hearing aid may not necessarily be of benefit. A copy of the Code of Practice should be made available on request, and this must be stated in any advertisement indicating that the dispenser is registered under the Hearing Aid Council Act.

Written information must be given for any trial, guarantee, service arrangements, financial and other relevant details, as outlined in the current Code of Practice, before a client is committed to, or supplied with, a hearing aid.

(e) Home visiting and exhibitions

Home visiting is strictly regulated except where the visit is requested by the client or an appropriate person acting on his or her behalf.

Where exhibitions are undertaken away from the permanent place of business, there must be adequate provision for after-care service and the full name and registered head office address must be prominently displayed.

(f) After-care

Service calls and complaints must always be dealt with promptly and efficiently.

The clauses that form the Code of Practice, which regulates dispensers of hearing aids, apply to all individuals who conduct or seek to conduct oral negotiations with a view to effecting the supply of a hearing aid for the use of a person with impaired hearing. The Code also regulates employers and trainees. All dispensers must therefore be conversant with the full current Code of Practice.

11.5 IMPROVING COMMUNICATIONS

11.5.1 COMMUNICATION

Even with normal hearing, a person will look at a speaker whenever possible to aid the communication process. In noisy situations there may be some reliance on mouth movements and facial expression to increase understanding.

With impaired hearing, there is likely to be some dependence on visual cues. Visual information may be through observing speech cues (speech-reading), or through a manual communication system (signing or finger-spelling). The degree of dependence is related to the degree of hearing impairment. Someone who is profoundly deaf is reliant on visual information, whereas with a mild loss hearing remains the primary communication channel.

11.5.2 SPEECH-READING

Speech-reading involves lip-reading together with observations of other visual cues, such as facial and hand movements.

Speech-reading is easier if the speaker:

- uses appropriate facial expressions and 'body language';
- uses a normal or slightly slowed rate of utterance;
- uses precise but not exaggerated articulation;
- is someone with whom the 'listener' is familiar;
- is positioned face to face at a distance of about 1.5 metres;
- does not cover the lips or smoke or chew while talking.

Many of the sounds of speech (phonemes) cannot be differentiated by the visual pattern alone. Groups of phonemes that look the same are known as a 'viseme'; for example, the bilabials 'p', 'b', 'm' form a viseme – a speech-reader could only conclude that one of that group had been spoken.

It is thought that only about 50% of a spoken message can be understood through lip-reading alone. Connected speech provides more information than visible articulatory movements alone (Chapter 4). When even significantly reduced hearing is coupled with speech-reading, the listener's ability to comprehend may be greatly increased.

Lip-reading classes provide activities to aid development of speech-reading. It is debatable whether or not lip-reading is a skill that can be taught, but in many cases classes provide graded practice and have the additional benefit of the more general group therapy.

11.5.3 AUDITORY TRAINING

An auditory training programme provides a series of exercises designed to develop listening skills and is most generally used for adults with a long-standing severe or profound hearing loss. Listening is more than just hearing, it requires active participation. The hearing impaired need to regain meaningful hearing and listening by practice and relearning over a period of time. The longer a hearing loss has been sustained, the longer will be the time needed for relearning, and auditory training may be very beneficial, particularly in difficult cases.

11.5.4 SPEECH THERAPY

We all normally use hearing to monitor our own voice; this is known as auditory feedback. Even a slight delay in hearing our own speech will cause us to stutter; this is demonstrated in the delayed feedback test sometimes used with non-organic deafness (section 12.4).

With impaired hearing there may also be a deterioration in speech and voice production, resulting in either poor articulation or an alteration of intensity level. If the loss is conductive, speech production is usually quieter. This is because the speaker's own voice sounds louder by bone conduction, while the voices of others and general background noises are all reduced because of the hearing loss.

If the loss is sensorineural, speech is usually louder as speakers cannot hear themselves or others, and often this is accompanied by poor consonant articulation since high frequency hearing is generally most affected.

Speech therapy may be provided to help maximize communication skills. The effect of congenital hearing loss on speech is more pronounced and the development of language may be delayed (Chapter 13).

11.6 THE ROLE OF OTHER SPECIALISTS

11.6.1 THE SOCIAL WORKER WITH DEAF PEOPLE

Social workers with deaf people undertake a specialist training in addition to that required for generic social work. This specialist training enables them to communicate and work effectively with deaf people. The role of these specialist social workers involves:

- maintaining a voluntary register of deaf (with and without speech) and hard of hearing people for the local authority;
- providing information to the deaf about statutory rights and entitlement to benefits;
- helping the deaf to resolve problems, whether these be physical, mental or financial.

Most of the time of social workers for deaf people is taken up with helping the profoundly prelingually deaf, whose main avenue of communication is sign language. This is a small minority group but communication difficulties compound their problems. Social workers may therefore find themselves acting as interpreters in court, hospital, at job interviews and so on, and dealing with discrimination at work or home.

11.6.2 HEARING THERAPISTS

Hearing therapists are generally hospital-based and work as part of a multidisciplinary team, which will include clinical and social work staff. The hearing therapist is involved in the rehabilitation of patients over the age of 16 with acquired hearing loss; they do not usually work with congenitally deaf people. The role is wide but includes the assessment of rehabilitative needs and the provision of programmes to maximize patients' communication skills. Such programmes may include instruction in the use of hearing aids and assistive devices, counselling, hearing tactics, lip-reading and auditory training. Hearing therapists undertake a one-year full-time course.

11.6.3 TEACHERS OF THE HEARING IMPAIRED

Teachers of the hearing impaired, more commonly called 'teachers of the deaf', are teachers who hold an additional certificate in education of the hearing impaired. This specialist qualification may be gained after the successful completion of a one-year full-time or equivalent part-time course. Teachers of the deaf are involved with children from diagnosis to the end of their education. Many are peripatetic, working with a caseload of children based in different schools rather than being based with a class or unit in one single school. Peripatetic teachers of the deaf usually spend part of their time working with the class or subject teachers (or the parents in the case of a pre-school child), rather than necessarily in the direct teaching of the hearing impaired child.

11.7 SUMMARY

The hearing aid audiologist can make a significant contribution to the hearing impaired client's quality of life. The provision of hearing aids is only part of an overall rehabilitative process that should answer certain questions:

- Is remediation necessary?
- Is amplification appropriate?
- What are the client's needs?
- Is medical referral necessary?
- What aids are needed?
- What counselling procedures are necessary?
- Has rehabilitation been successful?

The rehabilitation process may be handled entirely by the hearing aid audiologist, who must comply with the Hearing Aid Council Code of Practice, or it may involve a number of different specialists. The habilitation of children is undertaken by specialist teachers of the hearing impaired, while adult rehabilitation may involve a hearing therapist, within the health service. Ongoing support is provided for pre-lingually deaf adults by a social worker for the deaf.

REFERENCES

Ashley, J. (1991) The Silent House. *Being Deaf: The Experience of Deafness*, (eds G. Taylor and J. Bishop), The Open University, Milton Keynes.
British Standards Institution (1981) *BS 6083: Part 4, Hearing Aids: Specification for*

Magnetic Field Strength in Audio-frequency Induction Loops for Hearing Aid Purposes, British Standards Institution.

British Standards Institution (1988) *BS 2497: Part 5, Standard Reference Zero for the Calibration of Pure-Tone Air Conduction Audiometers*, British Standards Institution.

Goldstein, D.P. and Stevens, S.D.G. (1981) Audiological Rehabilitation: Management Model I. *Audiology*, **20**, 432–52.

Haggard, M.P., Gatehouse, S. and Davies, A.C. (1981) The High Prevalence of Hearing Disorders and its Implications for Services in the UK. *British Journal of Audiology*, **15**, 241–51.

Hallberg, L.R.–M. and Carlsson, S.G. (1991) Qualitative study of strategies for managing a hearing impairment. *British Journal of Audiology*, **25**(3), 201–11.

Hearing Aid Council (1990) *The Hearing Aid Council Code of Practice, Examinations and Registration*, The Hearing Aid Council, Milton Keynes.

Lutman, M.E., Brown, E.J. and Coles, R.R.A. (1987) Self-reported Disability and Handicap in the Population in Relation to Pure-Tone Threshold, Age, Sex and Type of Hearing Loss. *British Journal of Audiology*, **21**, 45–58.

Rendell, R.J., Williams, G., Vinton, M. and Croucher, L. (1992) Why Patients Choose to Purchase a Hearing Aid Privately. *British Journal of Audiology*, **26**(6), 325–7.

Tucker, I. and Nolan, M. (1984) *Educational Audiology*, Croom Helm, London.

Woolley, M. (1991) Acquired Hearing Loss: Acquired Oppression, in *Being Deaf: The Experience of Deafness* (eds G. Taylor and J. Bishop), The Open University, Milton Keynes.

FURTHER READING

Brooks, D.N. (1989) *Adult Aural Rehabilitation*, Chapman and Hall, London.

Davies, H. and Fallowfield, L. (1991) *Counselling and Communication in Health Care*, J. Wiley & Sons, Chichester.

Egan, G. (1990) *The Skilled Helper, Model Skills and Methods of Effective Helping*, 4th edn, Brooks Cole, Pacific Grove, California.

Pollack, M. (1988) *Amplification for the Hearing Impaired*, 3rd edn, Grune & Stratton, Orlando.

Sandlin, R.E. (1990) *Handbook of Hearing Aid Amplification*, Volume II, College-Hill Press, Boston.

PART THREE
Special Aspects of Hearing Aid Audiology

Assessment and management of special problems

12

12.1 TINNITUS

12.1.1 INTRODUCTION

Tinnitus is a relatively common complaint, which the Oxford Textbook of Medicine (1983) describes as:

> A sensation of noise in the ears or head. It may be related to disease of the cochlea or of the eighth nerve and can be produced by certain drugs of which quinine and the salicylates are the most important. It may be faint and perceived only in quiet surroundings, or it may be loud and continuous. It is variously described as a high-pitched whistling or hissing sound or occasionally as a low-pitched rumbling or machinery-like noise.

Research in this country suggests that over 17% of the population have had an experience of troublesome tinnitus, and that as many as 300 000 people in the UK have such severe tinnitus that they cannot work or function socially (Sheppard and Hawkridge, 1987). Tinnitus is always a symptom of some pathology and the first course of action must be the referral of the client for medical advice, in line with the Hearing Aid Council Code of Practice (1990). In the vast majority of cases there is no cure, and if medical and surgical treatment have been ruled out the hearing aid audiologist may try fitting maskers or hearing aids for relief from the tinnitus.

12.1.2 HEARING PROBLEMS AND TINNITUS

Tinnitus is frequently linked with hearing disorders and investigations may show a degree of similarity between the frequency of the tinnitus and that of the hearing loss. Where tinnitus accompanies a conductive loss it is most likely to be low frequency in nature (this also tends to be true of Menière's disorder). The tinnitus is often described as rumbling, humming or like the noise of machinery. Common causes include wax, fluid and otosclerosis. With the possible exception of the latter, medical treatment tends to be very effective for tinnitus which is linked with a conductive hearing problem.

Tinnitus more frequently accompanies sensorineural hearing loss and we still know relatively little about the mechanisms that may cause it. The current theory detailed below (Hazell, 1987) may help to explain some types of sensorineural tinnitus.

The outer, middle and inner ear concentrate sound energy to the hair cells in the cochlea. It is now thought that the organ of Corti is not a purely passive structure, but that it acts as a natural biomechanical hearing aid to focus sound energy efficiently on to the sensory hair cells. The inner hair cells appear to be passive receptors that fire the auditory nerve. The outer hair cells sharpen up the response of the basilar membrane, possibly utilizing:

- muscle proteins (actin and myosin, produced in the outer hair cells);
- the cuticular plate that surrounds the outer hair cells;
- the supporting cells of Deiters.

Selective stiffening of the basilar membrane actively sharpens the response, particularly to low intensity sounds. It may be that if the organ of Corti is damaged in one area, there is over-activity of the control mechanism, which may stimulate relatively healthy areas in close proximity. This could give rise to tinnitus, which would be close in frequency to the area of greatest hearing loss.

12.1.3 AIDS FOR THE RELIEF OF TINNITUS

There are a number of possible methods of treatment for tinnitus, including the use of drugs, surgery and electrical stimulation or utilizing cochlear implants for the profoundly deaf. The most common treatment, however, involves the use of masking instruments. These can be fitted by a hearing aid audiologist once medical and surgical intervention have been ruled out. Masking instruments do not 'cure' tinnitus, and counselling, methods of relaxation and the support of self-help groups can be important if success is to be achieved.

A tinnitus masker is a device, very similar to a hearing aid in appearance, which presents another, external, sound to the client. This other sound may fully or partially mask the tinnitus and some inhibition of the tinnitus may occur. Inhibition is the absence or reduction of the tinnitus after the masker is removed, and may last for only a few seconds or for much longer periods. Hearing aids can be used in combination with masking devices, or on their own. Hearing aids alone may provide some masking through the amplification of background noise, but they do not appear to achieve residual inhibition. We do not know enough about tinnitus to do more than speculate why maskers can be effective. It may be because they provide auditory masking, because of phase cancellation of the tinnitus sound, or perhaps because the masking noise restores 'balance' to the damaged part of the basilar membrane, reducing over-activity in adjacent areas. Whatever the reason, masking can, in many cases, be effective, although much rehabilitative counselling is usually needed. A correctly fitted masker, with or without a hearing aid as necessary, is the most effective method currently available for controlling sensorineural tinnitus.

12.1.4 TINNITUS ASSESSMENT

There are many ways of assessing tinnitus varying from recording the client's subjective account to lengthy simulations, perhaps involving use of a music synthesizer to match the frequency content. The methods used by hearing aid audiologists will reflect their equipment, personal interest and knowledge, and the time they have available. A reasonable match of the pitch and loudness of the client's tinnitus is important both for fitting and counselling. A more precise analysis of the nature of the sounds, while of interest, adds little of use to the fitting. An audiometer can be used quite successfully for tinnitus matching, although some tinnitus sufferers do find the matching test very difficult to perform.

The different stages involved in assessment (Figure 12.1) are as follows.

(a) Pure-tone audiometry

A not-masked pure-tone audiogram should be obtained prior to tinnitus matching. Uncomfortable loudness levels (ULLs) are important but should not be attempted at this stage because loud sounds may exacerbate tinnitus in a small proportion of cases.

(b) Pitch matching

A number of methods are available for pitch matching, but perhaps the most useful for the hearing aid audiologist's purposes is the adaptive

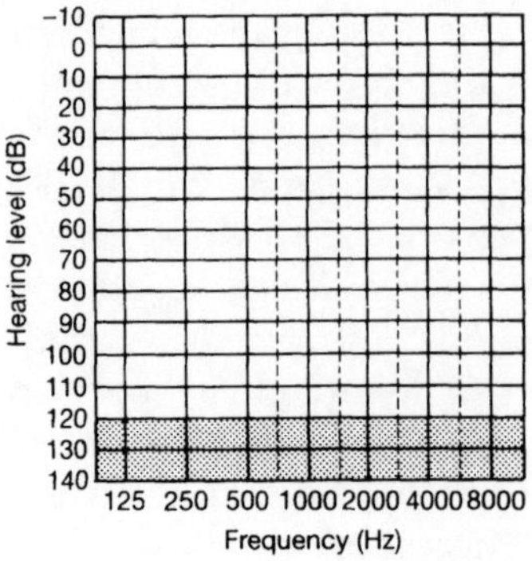

Hearing level (dB): -10, 0, 10, 20, 30, 40, 50, 60, 70, 80, 90, 100, 110, 120, 130, 140

Frequency (Hz): 125 250 500 1000 2000 4000 8000

Client Details:

Name:

Age:

Relevant History:

Masker/Aid Ordered:

TINNITUS EVALUATION

Pitch Matching   Audiometer used:

	Low frequency (below 1KHz)	Mid frequency (1-2KHz)	High frequency (above 2KHz)
Left	_____	_____	_____
Right	_____	_____	_____

Level Matching (dBHL)

Left Ear _____   Right Ear _____   Binaural _____

Test procedure: Loudness Balance to opposite ear _____
                 Loudness Balance to same ear   _____

Masking Evaluation

Type of audiometer or tinnitus masker used _____
Type of noise employed   _____
Masker control settings (if applicable)   _____

LEVELS REQUIRED (dBHL) TO MASK TINNITUS   UNCOMFORTABLE LEVELS

	L	R
Tinnitus Partially Masked		
Tinnitus Completely Masked		

Hz		250	500	1K	2K	6K	8K	Masking Noise
U L L	L							
	R							

Fig. 12.1 A suggested format for a tinnitus assessment form.

(bracketing) method. The client is asked to indicate whether his or her tinnitus is higher or lower in pitch than the test tone presented through the audiometer. A suitable explanation in layman's terms should be given, with examples or 'practice' as necessary.

Ideally the test tone should be presented in the same ear as that in which the tinnitus occurs, but in some cases it is necessary to test contralaterally. The tone should be introduced at one extreme of the available frequency range and at a level estimated to be comfortable. The selection of 8 kHz or 125 Hz is made on the basis of the client's description of his or her tinnitus. The tone should be presented for about 2 seconds, and repeated as necessary allowing time between presentations for the client to make the necessary comparison.

A practical example may help to clarify this. Suppose the client has described his tinnitus as a high-pitched noise, but when an 8 kHz tone is presented he describes the tinnitus as 'lower'. The next step is to present the lowest available frequency, usually 125 Hz. This time, the client describes his tinnitus as 'higher'. A 6 kHz frequency tone is presented next, and the extremes are gradually eliminated until the frequency, or frequency range, nearest to the tinnitus has been located.

Some clients confuse loudness with pitch. If this occurs, it may be necessary to perform some loudness matching at each frequency to be tested. Normally loudness matching is performed only at the frequency nearest that of the tinnitus.

(c) Loudness matching

A possible method for loudness matching is as follows. At the frequency matched as the nearest to the pitch of the tinnitus, the tone is presented initially at threshold (based on the audiogram). The tone should be held for 2 seconds, and increased in 5 dB steps until the client judges it to be of equal loudness to the tinnitus.

It is important to realize that severe tinnitus may appear very quiet when matched to external sounds. Levels as low in intensity as 10 dB above threshold can be perceived as being very severe, perhaps because of its inescapability or possibly due in part to the effects of recruitment.

(d) Masking evaluation

An indication of the likely benefit of masking may be obtained using wide band masking noise from the audiometer; alternatively narrow band masking or pure-tones may be used. The aim is to find the minimal level of masking that is effective. The masking noise is introduced at or below threshold and increased in 5 dB steps until the client indicates he or she can no longer hear the tinnitus. At each step, the noise should be held for 5 seconds. This is followed by a rest period of a further 5 seconds so that the client can again hear the tinnitus. When the minimal masking level (MML) has been found, it is maintained for up to 3 minutes. If, during this time, the tinnitus becomes audible again, the masking noise may be raised in 5 dB steps until it becomes effective once more.

The difference between the initial level and the level required after 3 minutes will indicate the masking decay. Where masking decays, it may be necessary to amend the aim of masking therapy, to effect partial masking for the client. 'Chasing' the tinnitus is not usually helpful and may result in high levels of masking noise being used. Generally, masking may be effective at low intensity levels, and the lower the level at which it is effective, the more likely it is to be accepted by the client.

(e) Uncomfortable loudness level (ULL)

ULLs must be obtained after all tinnitus investigations are completed, because loud sounds may heighten the tinnitus. If loud sounds do have this effect, the output of a hearing aid may be adjusted to minimize the problem, utilizing peak clipping, or automatic gain control as necessary. Testing for the ULLs is carried out according to the British Society of Audiology recommended method (1987), but ULLs must be found for the masking noise as well as the audiometric frequencies tested.

12.1.5 THE REHABILITATION PROGRAMME

The ideal tinnitus programme, which can be offered by a hearing aid audiologist after the client has obtained medical advice, will include:

- consultation, assessment and impressions;
- fitting;
- follow-up, e.g. after one month or sooner;
- further appointments as necessary for rehabilitation;
- further audiometry, e.g. bi-annually, if high levels of masking are used or there is a progressive element to the hearing loss.

(a) Consultation, assessment and impressions

Tinnitus frequently causes stress, anxiety and poor concentration. Clients may feel their tinnitus impairs their ability to hear clearly. Often this is due to an associated hearing loss, rather than the tinnitus itself. Careful history-taking and assessment are important. The assessment will provide an indication of the possible benefit of masking but, as with hearing aids, benefit may be greatest after a period of time has allowed the client to adjust to its use. The ideal is always to facilitate a trial period with hearing aids or maskers. Where tinnitus is bilateral, two instruments will often be required. Even where the tinnitus is monaural, there are some cases in which bilateral masking is still required.

Impressions should be taken for both ears and the ear moulds obtained should be of the skeleton open ear type or have a vent that is as large as possible. Solid moulds tend to increase the effect of the tinnitus by occlusion.

(b) Fitting

If a combination hearing aid and masker is used it is customary to fit the instrument as a hearing aid first. Masking is switched on at the lowest volume and raised until it is at threshold. It is then increased in small increments until the lowest intensity sufficient to just render the tinnitus inaudible is found. The lowest effective intensity should always be used. If tinnitus breaks through, it may be necessary to counsel the client to regard the masking as a distraction rather than relief. A masker that is adjustable by the audiologist permits trial with low, mid- and high frequency noise to establish which is most effective. A frequency similar to the tinnitus may be most effective in inhibiting the tinnitus, but in many cases the most effective masking noise is lower in frequency than the tinnitus. Selection of the noise to use generally involves an element of trial and error.

The client needs to be instructed in the techniques of use, most of which are very similar to instructions for use of a hearing aid. The use of a masker, as of a hearing aid, is built up gradually. The client should be advised that, while a hearing aid may be used continuously, masking should be used only as much as required. A schedule for its use can be discussed with the client, for instance a period of masking at night is often helpful in relaxing the client ready for sleep. Other advice should include a recommendation to avoid loud sounds and to reduce intake of caffeine, alcohol and aspirin, since these can worsen tinnitus. Total abstinence, at least during the period of adjustment to masking, is the ideal.

(c) Follow-up

Hearing aid audiologists are well acquainted with the need for follow-up to establish the effective use of hearing aids. Counselling and support, often over a prolonged period, are even more crucial to the tinnitus client. Thorough rehabilitation should be normal practice for new users of both hearing aids and masking instruments.

Masking has not been shown to cause any deterioration in hearing (Hazell, 1985), but if high levels are used, or if there is a progressive element to the hearing loss, it is prudent to carry out regular hearing checks.

12.1.6 SUMMARY

Tinnitus can be a troublesome condition from which some relief may be achieved through the use of masking instruments. Assessment and fitting are important aspects of the tinnitus programme, but support and counselling are also very necessary to the vast majority of clients. The success of masking instrument use varies widely, and success depends heavily on the techniques used by the hearing aid audiologist.

REFERENCES FOR SECTION 12.1

British Society of Audiology (1987) Recommended Method for Uncomfortable Loudness Level (ULL). *British Journal of Audiology*, **21**, 231.
Hazell, J.W.P. (1985) Management of Tinnitus: Discussion Paper. *Journal of Royal Society of Medicine*, **78**, 56–60.
Hazell, J.W.P. (1987) *Tinnitus*, Churchill Livingstone, Edinburgh.
Hearing Aid Council (1990) *The Hearing Aid Council Code of Practice, Examinations and Registration*, Hearing Aid Council, Milton Keynes.
Oxford Textbook of Medicine (1983) (eds D.J. Weatherall, J.G.G. Ledingham and D.A. Warrell), Oxford University Press, Oxford.
Sheppard, L. and Hawkridge, A. (1987) *Tinnitus – Learning to Live with it*, Ashgrove Press, Bath.

FURTHER READING FOR SECTION 12.1

Coles, R., Davis, A. and Smith, P. (1990) Tinnitus: Its Epidemiology and Management, in *Presbyacusis and other Age-Related Aspects*, J.H. Jensen (ed.), 14th Danavox Symposium, Copenhagen.
Feldmann, H. (ed.) (1987) Proceedings of III International Tinnitus Seminar, 1987, Münster, Germany. Harsch Verlag Karlsruhe, Münster, pp. 121–8.
Hazell, J. (1987) *Tinnitus*, Churchill Livingstone, Edinburgh.

12.2 IMPEDANCE AUDIOMETRY

12.2.1 INTRODUCTION

The role of the conductive pathway is to convey sound energy efficiently to the cochlea. If the sound wave finds it easy to set the eardrum into vibration, much energy is passed on and only a little is reflected. However, if it is difficult to set the eardrum into vibration, much energy is reflected. The difficulty or hindrance to the flow of energy is called **impedance**. The impedance at the eardrum tells us how well the middle ear is functioning. The aim of impedance measurements is to assess the efficiency of the middle ear mechanism at passing on sound energy.

12.2.2 THE MIDDLE EAR AND ACOUSTIC IMPEDANCE

When a sound wave reaches the eardrum some of the energy sets the drum vibrating and some is reflected. The eardrum movements are carried by the ossicles in the middle ear to the cochlea. The function of the middle ear is to act as a transformer, between the low pressure required to transmit sound through air and the relatively high pressure needed to transmit sound through the perilymph in the cochlea. In essence, the middle ear increases the pressure reaching the cochlea. This is achieved mainly by concentrating the sound energy arriving at the eardrum on to the much smaller stapes footplate. This is not unlike the effect of a stiletto heel (Figure 12.2), which concentrates the weight of the body on to a small area such that it may make a mark on the floor whereas a larger heel area does not have the same effect. In the middle ear, there is a small additional effect from the lever action of the ossicles, and a slight improvement, especially in the higher frequencies, due to the conical shape of the eardrum.

Normally this system is very efficient and only a little sound is reflected by the eardrum. The major part of the sound energy is transformed into powerful vibrations to stimulate the cochlea. However, if the middle ear system is altered, for example as a result of disease, the proportion of sound transmitted through it may alter. The efficiency of the system is reduced and more energy is lost either by reflection from the eardrum or friction in the middle ear. Consequently less sound reaches the cochlea and the patient experiences a 'conductive' hearing loss.

The acoustic impedance of the middle ear is the term used to describe the resistance presented by the middle ear to the passage of sound.

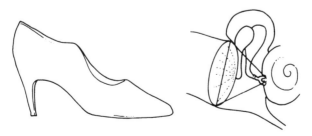

Fig. 12.2 The transformer action of the middle ear is similar in concept to the effect of a stiletto heel.

This varies according to the frequency of the sound passing through, and at high frequency the impedance is mainly due to the mass of the three bones. However, at low frequencies the acoustic impedance is mainly due to the stiffness of the eardrum and the ossicular chain. In most conductive conditions, the middle ear system becomes less mobile and the stiffness of the eardrum is increased. A greater than normal proportion of the acoustic energy is reflected by the stiffened eardrum and a smaller than usual proportion is passed on to the cochlea.

Investigations into the proportion of sound reflected by the eardrum can give information about the acoustic impedance of the ear.

12.2.3 THE CONCEPT OF IMPEDANCE

Impedance in audiometry is simply the difficulty or hindrance to the flow of acoustic energy along the conductive pathway. Compliance or admittance is, conversely, the mobility or acceptance of the system.

Impedance is not difficult to conceptualize. When you move a cricket bat through air it moves easily, but you would have to apply far more force to make the same stroke in a swimming pool. This is because air is a low impedance medium and water is a high impedance medium.

A similar principle applies in the ear, where acoustic energy has to move from air to the liquid-filled inner ear. Only if the impedance of the two mediums are matched, will energy pass readily from one medium to the other. Impedance can be viewed as being influenced by the resistance of the system and the way it reacts (that is, its reactance).

Resistance removes energy from the system and converts it to another form, as in friction, for example, between the joints of the ossicles. This is a very small component of the impedance of the middle ear.

Reactance is made up of two elements, stiffness and inertia. The inertia of the system relates mainly to the mass of the ossicles and is of consequence for higher frequency sounds above about 1.5 kHz.

Although the proportion of energy accepted or rejected by the middle ear is the result of a complex interaction of the three elements that make it up, only stiffness is of clinical importance.

Impedance = resistance + reactance (made up of stiffness and inertia)

Disorders of the conductive hearing mechanism generally cause changes in stiffness. Stiffness, like inertia, is frequency-dependent. Stiffness dominates in the low frequency region.

12.2.4 PRINCIPLES AND EQUIPMENT

The electro-acoustic impedance bridge, or admittance meter, is an instrument that provides information on the functioning of the middle ear. Impedance is resistance to the flow of energy, while admittance is the efficiency of the system to absorb such energy. The term 'immitance' is sometimes used to mean the clinical application of impedance or admittance, but it is not a preferred term.

Two tests widely used in audiometry are:

1. tympanometry;
2. acoustic reflex measurement.

Each is an objective measure requiring little if any co-operation from the subject; both are quick, easy and non-invasive and are thus applicable to every age group, from babies to the oldest of senior citizens, and every degree of hearing loss.

12.2.5 TYMPANOMETRY

For the purposes of tympanometry a small probe made up of three tubes (Figure 12.3) is sealed in the ear canal using a small plastic cuff or tip. The first tube carries a continuous low frequency probe tone, which is passed into the ear canal by the miniature receiver. The second tube monitors the sound level and the third tube allows the pressure in the outer ear to be altered and measured.

Tympanometry is the measurement of eardrum compliance as the air pressure is altered in the external ear canal. The eardrum is most compliant, that is, it moves most freely, when the air pressure in the middle ear is the same as that in the ear canal. This would normally be at atmospheric pressure, but for the purposes of tympanometry, the ear canal is blocked and the air pressure in the canal is artificially varied. When the pressure equalizes with that of the middle ear and the eardrum moves most freely, sound energy passes readily through the eardrum with little reflected. The level of reflected sound in the ear

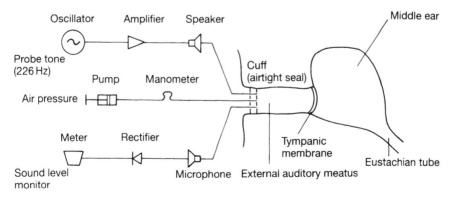

Fig. 12.3 An electro-acoustic impedance meter.

canal is recorded, and will be at its lowest at the point of maximum compliance.

Patients are usually told that the tympanogram is a record of how the eardrum moves, although it is really a graph showing how the SPL in the outer ear changes as the air pressure alters. From this we can draw conclusions about the mobility of the middle ear system. The compliance or mobility of the ear is usually expressed in cubic centimetres (cc) of equivalent volume.

Sound pressure level is a function of a closed cavity volume. With a known probe tone, which in tympanometry is usually a 226 Hz tone at 65 dBSPL, the SPL will decrease as the cavity size increases. The compliance of the middle ear is therefore expressed as an equivalent cavity volume. The intensity of the probe tone is such that it will not produce a reflex contraction of the stapedius muscles.

The procedure followed in tympanometry can be summarized in a series of steps:

1. The probe in the cuff is inserted into the ear canal so that an airtight seal is achieved.
2. The middle ear canal pressure is altered between +200 and −400 decapascals (daPa) or millimetres of water (mm H_2O). (1 daPa $\simeq$ 1 mm H_2O).
3. Compliance of the eardrum is measured as the relative change in sound pressure level in the ear canal, as the air pressure is increased and decreased.
4. When the sound waves strike the eardrum, some of the energy will be reflected. If the eardrum is stiff, more of the energy will be reflected, causing a greater SPL in the cavity.
5. Tympanometry starts with an increase in air pressure in the canal (+200 daPa), which pushes the eardrum so that it cannot move freely. Much sound is therefore reflected and a high SPL recorded.
6. The pressure is reduced and, as the eardrum begins to move more freely, little sound is reflected and a low SPL is recorded.
7. The point of maximum compliance occurs when the lowest SPL is recorded in the ear canal.
8. At the point of maximum compliance, middle ear pressure will be equal to the pressure in the ear canal.
9. Compliance is measured in cc of equivalent canal volume. A much larger than normal static canal volume can identify a perforated eardrum.

12.2.6 CHARACTERISTICS OF THE TYMPANOGRAM

Two characteristics of the tympanogram are of interest:

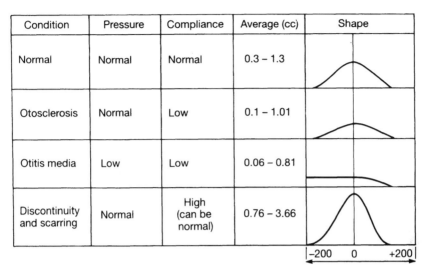

Condition	Pressure	Compliance	Average (cc)	Shape
Normal	Normal	Normal	0.3 – 1.3	
Otosclerosis	Normal	Low	0.1 – 1.01	
Otitis media	Low	Low	0.06 – 0.81	
Discontinuity and scarring	Normal	High (can be normal)	0.76 – 3.66	−200 0 +200

Fig. 12.4 Typical tympanogram configurations likely to be seen in a clinical population. Values of compliance from 0.3 cc to 1.3 cc obtained at a pressure between +30 daPa and −80 daPa are considered to be within the normal range.

1. its shape;
2. the air pressure at maximum compliance.

The shape, rather than any absolute value, of the tympanogram is most important because wide variations occur within the various pathologies, and only the overall pattern is useful.

Common shapes related to certain ear conditions are reasonably easy to recognize by comparison with the shape of an average normal tympanogram. For example, if a client has fluid in the middle ear the eardrum will not move freely at any point and the resultant shape is a flat graph indicating high impedance. Where low pressure, without fluid, is present in the middle ear the normal curve is displaced, and such a condition may be responsible for slight 'unexplained' conductive hearing loss. If the ear is perforated or a grommet is in place it will be impossible to maintain pressure unless the Eustachian tube is blocked; in this case the cavity volume will be abnormally large and the graph will be very flat. Some common shapes are shown in Figure 12.4.

12.2.7 THE ACOUSTIC REFLEX

The middle ear has two muscles. The stapedius muscle is approximately 6 mm long and is located in a vertical hole in the bulge in the posterior wall of the middle ear, known as the pyramidal fossa. It is attached to the neck of the stapes by a tendon that is about 2 mm long. On contraction it pulls the stapes outwards and backwards, which stiffens the ossicular chain, increasing the acoustic impedance. The nerve controlling the stapedius muscle is the seventh cranial (facial) nerve. The tensor tympani muscle is about 20 mm long and lies in a bony canal alongside the Eustachian tube. It passes around a bony ledge before being attached to the upper part of the handle of the malleus by a 6 mm tendon. It is controlled by the fifth cranial (trigeminal) nerve, which is mainly responsible for reporting sensation over the face. When the muscle contracts, it tends to pull the malleus forward and inward to stiffen the ossicular chain. The acoustic reflex is mainly the result of the stapedius muscles' contraction, and it is therefore often referred to as the stapedial reflex. Very loud sounds may cause a startle response that will involve the tensor tympani. When the muscles contract, low frequencies are attenuated by up to 20 dB. The function of the reflex is not certain, but it is probable that its main purpose is to filter out the most intense sounds in one's own speech. It also has a protective function, but this is probably a by-product.

A loud sound, usually 70 to 90 dB above threshold, in either ear will cause a reflex contraction of both left and right stapedius muscles. This causes a slight increase in acoustic impedance. The acoustic reflex test is a measure of the threshold at which the stapedial reflex occurs. The acoustic reflex threshold for pure-tones is higher than the reflex threshold for white noise. Acoustic reflexes can be measured ipsilaterally (in the same ear) or contralaterally (in the opposite ear) because a signal applied to one ear causes a reflex contraction in both ears. The threshold of the tone used to elicit the reflex is always recorded for the ear to which the tone is presented. This is known as the stimulated ear.

In order for an acoustic reflex to be obtained, the patient must:

- perceive a 'loud' sound;
- have a normal middle ear on the measuring probe side (the reflex response produces a **small** increase in impedance; if the eardrum already has a high impedance due to glue ear, for example, the reflex response will not be noticed);
- have an intact reflex arc (Figure 12.5).

A reflex becomes less likely if there is a conductive hearing loss. A conductive loss of 25 dB in the stimulated ear will usually abolish the reflex. A conductive loss of only 10 dB in the probe ear may prevent the reflex from being recorded, because the eardrum is already stiffened.

The acoustic reflex indicates the loudness of the signal. A conductive loss of 25 dB or more is likely to prevent the patient from perceiving the signal as sufficiently loud to elicit the acoustic reflex. However, in the case of cochlear pathology, the patient often hears the sound as if it

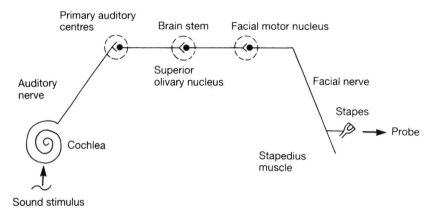

Fig. 12.5 The stapedial reflex arc.

were much louder, due to recruitment. The acoustic reflex threshold then occurs at less than the normal 70 dB to 90 dB above the threshold of hearing. The gap between the threshold of hearing and the reflex threshold is known as the span. Where there is a cochlear disorder, an acoustic reflex may occur with a span of less than 60 dB.

A low acoustic reflex threshold is a simple objective test to identify a cochlear disorder. With a cochlear hearing loss of 60 dB or less there is a 90% chance of observing an acoustic reflex. Naturally, as the hearing loss increases, the chance of observing a reflex decreases. However, when such a reflex does occur it indicates severe recruitment.

Reflex thresholds have little value on their own but aid diagnosis in conjunction with other results. A span between the threshold of hearing and the reflex threshold of 60 dB or less indicates a cochlear loss; while a difference of greater than 15 dB between the reflex threshold of each ear may suggest a problem beyond the cochlea, that is, a retrocochlear disorder.

If hearing thresholds have not been obtained, perhaps due to a severe loss in a young child, or a non-organic problem, reflex thresholds can be used to confirm that hearing is present at that level. Reflexes may also be used to suggest an appropriate uncomfortable loudness level where one cannot otherwise be obtained, as discomfort usually occurs approximately 10 dB above the acoustic reflex.

12.2.8 SUMMARY

The role of the conductive pathway is to convey sound energy efficiently to the cochlea. The tympanic membrane and ossicular chain present an impedance to incoming sound waves. At low frequencies, the impedance is governed principally by the stiffness of the system. Most causes of conductive hearing loss affect the stiffness of the middle ear. If the stiffness can be measured it can provide valuable information about conditions of the middle ear. The function of tympanometry is to measure how the impedance alters with variation in air pressure in the ear canal. The shape of the compliance curve and the value of the middle ear pressure can be of great assistance in pin-pointing the nature of a middle ear disorder.

An acoustic reflex is normally obtained at 70 dB to 90 dB above hearing threshold level. A sound stimulus applied to one ear will cause a bilateral reflex. A conductive loss in either ear reduces the likelihood of obtaining a reflex. Where there is a sensorineural hearing loss of cochlear origin, an acoustic reflex is likely to be present at sensation levels of 60 dB or less. This is because the acoustic threshold indicates the subjective loudness of a sound, not the objective intensity. Recruitment is present with most, if not all, cochlear disorders and a reduced reflex threshold is therefore likely to be obtained.

FURTHER READING FOR SECTION 12.2

Arlinger, S. (1989) *Manual of Practical Audiometry*, Volume I, Whurr Publishers, London.

British Society of Audiology (1992) Recommended Procedure for Tympanometry. *British Journal of Audiology*, **26**, 255–7.

Jerger, J. (1980) *Clinical Impedance Audiometry*, American Electromedics Corporation, Massachusetts.

Tucker, I. and Nolan, M. (1984) *Educational Audiology*, Croom Helm, London.

12.3 SPECIALIZED AUDIOMETRIC TESTS

12.3.1 INTRODUCTION

Conductive hearing loss can be separated from sensorineural loss relatively easily using pure-tone audiometry, but to differentiate the various types of sensorineural hearing loss is more difficult.

A number of specialized audiometric tests are used to distinguish sensory (or cochlear) from neural (or retrocochlear) hearing disorders. These tests can provide powerful clues to the site and probable cause of sensorineural hearing loss.

Individual test results are not always reliable and the results of a number of different audiometric tests are normally used in conjunction with information revealed from the case history and physical examination. Information that may help to distinguish cochlear disorders from those which occur beyond the cochlea, or retrocochlear, may be obtained from acoustic reflex measurement, speech audiometry, Békèsy audiometry (section 12.5.2) and electric response audiometry. There is also a number of specialized audiometric tests that are used routinely in many clinics to aid diagnosis. These include the Short Increment Sensitivity Index (SISI) test, the Alternate Binaural Loudness Balance (ABLB) test and tests of auditory adaptation or tone decay.

12.3.2 TESTS OF COCHLEAR FUNCTION

(a) The Alternate Binaural Loudness Balance (ABLB) test

In the normal ear a linear relationship exists between an increase in intensity and the related increase in perceived loudness. However, when damage has occurred in the hair cells of the cochlea, a loss of hearing sensitivity may be accompanied by an abnormality known as recruitment, in which the subjective sensation of loudness builds up at a more rapid rate than normal. For patients with recruitment, a small increase in intensity will produce an abnormally large increase in the subjective sensation of loudness.

This abnormal growth in loudness is subjective and therefore cannot be directly measured. In cases of unilateral loss, the normal ear can be used as a reference for comparison. The Alternate Binaural Loudness Balance (ABLB) test compares loudness growth in the abnormal ear with loudness growth in the normal ear. There is no single recognized procedure and the following is an outline of one test method that may be used.

A tone, 20 dB above the air conduction threshold, is introduced in the good ear and held for 1 second. A tone of the same frequency and estimated to be of equal loudness is introduced to the poorer ear and also held for 1 second. The tone is presented to each ear alternately and the intensity in the poorer ear is raised or lowered until the patient indicates that the tone in each ear is equally loud. This balancing continues at 20 dB intervals in the good ear until full recruitment is reached or the test is discontinued, either because discomfort is experienced, or because the maximum output of the audiometer has been reached.

The test is performed at one or more frequencies, usually 1 kHz or 2 kHz and 4 kHz. The results may be plotted on a laddergram, in which case, at each level tested, points are joined to illustrate sounds of equal loudness. Laddergrams are helpful in understanding the principle of the ABLB test, but graphs are most generally used to plot results in clinical practice. If, as in Figure 12.6, the left ear shows a hearing loss of 40 dB, a 40 dBHL tone will sound the same as a 0 dBHL tone in the normal ear. Taking these thresholds as a base line, any increase in intensity added identically to both left and right ears results in tones

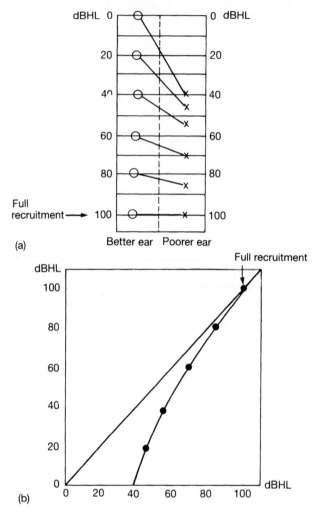

Fig. 12.6 Results of an ABLB test plotted both as a laddergram (a) and as a graph (b).

that are heard as equally loud in both ears. This is normal loudness growth. In cases of recruitment an increase in intensity, applied identically to both ears, may appear as a much louder increase in the impaired ear. Full recruitment is a symptom of cochlear damage. It is possible for loudness to increase so rapidly that, beyond a certain intensity, a tone may appear louder to the poorer ear than it does to the better ear. This is known as hyper-recruitment. Where the damage to the ear is retrocochlear almost any pattern of loudness growth may occur, including derecruitment. Derecruitment is where loudness grows

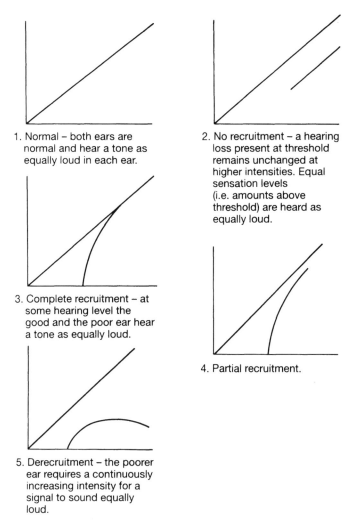

1. Normal – both ears are normal and hear a tone as equally loud in each ear.

2. No recruitment – a hearing loss present at threshold remains unchanged at higher intensities. Equal sensation levels (i.e. amounts above threshold) are heard as equally loud.

3. Complete recruitment – at some hearing level the good and the poor ear hear a tone as equally loud.

4. Partial recruitment.

5. Derecruitment – the poorer ear requires a continuously increasing intensity for a signal to sound equally loud.

Fig. 12.7 Some possible outcomes of the ABLB test.

more slowly than normal, and is most often found with eighth nerve damage. Some possible patterns of loudness growth are shown in Figure 12.7.

A two-channel audiometer is required for the ABLB test, which may be carried out manually or automatically. The procedure is only really useful if the loss is unilateral. When the loss is bilateral, but each ear has normal hearing at some frequency, a monaural loudness balancing test can be attempted. This compares the loudness of a low frequency tone with the loudness of a higher frequency tone in the same ear. The intensity is raised in 10 dB steps using a method similar to that in the ABLB test. However, judgement of equal loudness between different frequencies is much more difficult for the patient.

(b) The Short Increment Sensitivity Index (SISI)

Small changes in intensity cannot normally be detected at near threshold levels. Several decibels change in intensity are required before the listener can detect any change in loudness. As the tone becomes louder, small changes are much easier to detect. This is true for all listeners. The smallest change that can be detected is termed the difference limen for intensity. Very small changes in intensity at near threshold levels can only be detected in cochlear disorders. Both loudness recruitment and the ability to hear very small changes in intensity may be observed in cases of cochlear damage.

The Short Increment Sensitivity Index (SISI) is designed to test the patient's ability to detect 1 dB changes in intensity superimposed on a tone presented 20 dB above threshold. The SISI test indicates the presence of cochlear damage but is not a direct indication of the presence of recruitment.

A continuous tone is introduced at 20 dB above threshold. Every 5 seconds the tone rises by 1 dB and this rise is held for one-fifth of a second (Figure 12.8). The patient signals whenever he or she hears a rise in the tone. After 20 rises in the tone have been presented the patient's score is multiplied by five to obtain a percentage. Patients with normal hearing, middle ear or retrocochlear disorders obtain very low scores, whereas patients with cochlear disorders usually score very highly. Typically, normal hearing, middle ear or retrocochlear disorders score between 0% and 30%, and cochlear disorders score between 70% and 100%. The higher the SISI score, the more likely it is that the pathology is cochlear. Frequencies tested are usually 1 kHz and 4 kHz, because lower frequencies are less likely to show positive results.

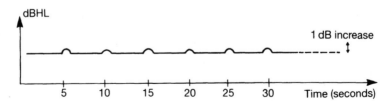

Fig. 12.8 The SISI test: every 5 seconds the tone presented jumps by 1 dB. This is repeated 20 times.

(c) Tests of auditory adaptation

It is a normal phenomenon of hearing that sounds appear loudest when they are first heard. A signal held for some time will appear to fade, or decay. Extremely rapid tone decay may indicate a retrocochlear disorder. Retrocochlear hearing loss can be due to damage anywhere from the eighth nerve to the brain. Retrocochlear disorders are relatively rare, but they may be very serious in nature.

Several procedures exist for quantifying tone decay. In 1957, Carhart reported a tone decay technique that is still in use today. However, Carhart's tone decay test is time-consuming, and a modified version of it, proposed by Rosenberg, is more widely used in clinical practice. The Rosenberg modified procedure (1969) is carried out as follows.

A tone is introduced at 5 dB above threshold and the patient is asked to signal whenever the tone disappears. Every time the tone fades and becomes inaudible, the intensity is raised by 5 dB. The test continues for 1 minute. At the end of this time, the degree of tone decay is expressed as the number of decibels by which the tone has been raised. Decay is considered significant if the tone has had to be raised by 20 dB or more. Extreme tone decay of over 30 dB is often found in eighth nerve pathology, although it can also be present with some cochlear disorders. It is usual to test at two or more frequencies, as decay is sometimes more marked at one frequency than another. The frequencies most often used are 2 kHz and 500 Hz, or 1 kHz and 4 kHz.

Retrocochlear disorders can be life-threatening, and as tone decay can be used to provide a screening test for retrocochlear pathology it is useful to include in a battery of clinical tests.

12.3.3 SUMMARY

Pure-tone thresholds provide a great deal of information about hearing loss, including the separation of conductive from sensorineural disorders. Specialized tests are used to provide further information on the location of the damage within the auditory system. A number of specialized audiometric tests exists.

Alternate Binaural Loudness Balance (ABLB) tests for recruitment in cases of unilateral hearing loss, by comparing the growth of loudness in the impaired ear with that in the normal ear. The Short Increment Sensitivity Index (SISI) determines the patient's ability to detect very small changes in intensity at near threshold levels. Tests of tone decay consider the degree to which audibility is lost when the ear is continuously stimulated with a pure-tone at near threshold levels.

These tests help in the differentiation between cochlear and retrocochlear hearing losses. The tests described are examples of those that may be used. They are not infallible diagnostic indicators and are not intended to be used on their own. Clinical diagnosis consists of applying a number or 'battery' of tests, and the results of specialized diagnostic tests are interpreted in the light of information provided during pure-tone threshold tests and the case history.

REFERENCES FOR SECTION 12.3

Carhart, R. (1957) Clinical determination of abnormal auditory adaptation. *Archives of Otolaryngology*, **65**, 32–9.
Rosenberg, P.E. (1969) *Tone Decay*, Maico Audiological Library Series, Report 6.

FURTHER READING FOR SECTION 12.3

Arlinger, S. (1989) *Manual of Practical Audiometry*, Volume I, Whurr Publishers, London.
Jacobsen, J.T. and Northern, J.L. (1991) *Diagnostic Audiology*, Pro-ed, Austen.
Katz, J. (1985) *Handbook of Clinical Audiology*, 3rd edn., Williams & Wilkins, Baltimore.
Martin, F. (1991) *An Introduction to Audiology*, Prentice Hall, New Jersey.

12.4 NON-ORGANIC HEARING LOSS

12.4.1 INTRODUCTION

Non-organic hearing loss refers to a condition in which there is no apparent organic (bodily) disorder to explain the hearing problem. Non-organic hearing loss is also known as functional loss or pseudo-hypacusis. These are general terms that can be used to describe an apparent hearing loss which may be either psychogenic (genuine) or malingering (false).

12.4.2 PSYCHOGENIC HEARING LOSS

Psychogenic hearing loss is genuine but of psychological origin. It is usually due to hysteria and at one time was termed 'hysterical deafness'. This kind of hearing loss is usually bilateral and profound; it persists even in sleep and the special tests for non-organic hearing loss are unlikely to provide much useful information.

12.4.3 MALINGERING

Malingering is the deliberate faking of a hearing loss for gain, most commonly for compensation purposes. Many malingerers do have a genuine hearing loss but exaggerate the loss to increase their claim. Routine audiometry is of little value in obtaining correct thresholds, but there are signs that should alert the audiologist to the possibility of non-organic loss. The patient's behaviour may raise suspicions, for instance if the patient exaggerates their reliance on lip-reading, and test results are often inconsistent. A patient may have excellent speech discrimination despite a hearing loss that seems severe, or there may be no evidence of cross-hearing in an apparent unilateral hearing loss.

It is not uncommon for children to manifest non-organic hearing loss under certain circumstances. The attention centred on them and the excuse the loss provides may help a child to overcome problems that are unrelated to a hearing difficulty. The audiologist must establish true thresholds but should take care to obtain further investigation and treatment for the child's underlying problems if this is required (Brooks and Geoghegan, 1992).

Special 'attention raising' techniques are often used to obtain true thresholds. These are very simple, for example a child may be asked to say 'yes' when he or she hears a tone and 'no' when he or she does not. Many children will say 'no' to presented tones that are below their feigned threshold. As long as the audiologist is sure no visual or timing clues have been given, true thresholds may be obtained in this way. Older and more sophisticated children are less easy to deceive but often it is unnecessary to use the more complex tests required to ascertain true thresholds for the adult. Many (adult) tests for non-organic hearing loss exist; some are listed below.

(a) Repeat pure-tone threshold tests

Many adults are unable to provide consistent false audiograms. If the thresholds on repeat tests vary by more than 10 dB, non-organic hearing loss may be suspected. (Children are often much better at maintaining consistent non-organic audiometric thresholds. This test is therefore unsuitable for children.)

(b) The Lombard test

This test is based on the principle that a normally hearing person will raise his or her voice in the presence of background noise. The patient is asked to read aloud and, at some unannounced time, masking noise is introduced and gradually increased in intensity. If the hearing loss is genuine, the noise will have no effect until it at least exceeds the deafness. If the hearing loss is fake, the patient may raise his or her voice without realizing it.

(c) Doerfler-Stewart test

It is usually possible to respond to speech even when masking noise is 10 dB to 15 dB greater than the intensity of the speech signals. The patient with a non-organic loss often assumes that any level of masking noise should prevent the hearing of speech. If a speech test is presented with masking, the non-organic patient will stop repeating words, sometimes even when the noise is less intense than the speech signal. A positive test suggests a non-organic loss but does not reveal the true threshold levels.

(d) Delayed speech feedback test

It is normal for speakers to monitor their own voice unconsciously as they speak, using their own hearing. If this auditory feedback mechanism is disturbed, speech is affected. This test involves the use of a tape recorder that has separate record and playback heads. The patient's voice is recorded as he or she speaks and played back with a very slight delay of 0.1 to 0.2 seconds. The creation of delayed feedback disturbs the speaker's speech pattern, causing slowing, stuttering or other difficulty. If the hearing loss is genuine, delayed feedback at intensities below threshold will have no effect on the speech.

(e) The Stenger test

This test is the most widely used to identify monaural non-organic hearing loss. It employs the principle that, where two tones of the same frequency are presented simultaneously, only the most intense one is heard.

A two-channel audiometer is used to introduce a tone 10 dB above the threshold of the 'better' ear. The patient should respond. A tone is then presented to the 'deaf' ear 10 dB below its given threshold. Tones are presented simultaneously to both ears, 10 dB above the threshold of the better ear, and 10 dB below the threshold of the 'deaf' ear.

A patient with a genuine hearing loss will continue to respond to the tone that is 10 dB above threshold in the better ear. If the patient does not respond, this is because he or she can only hear the tone in the 'deaf' ear, which he or she refuses to admit. The patient can only hear the loudest tone and does not realize there is still a tone above threshold in the 'better' ear.

The test can be continued to reveal approximate true thresholds. For instance, the tone is presented at 10 dBHL above the threshold of the better ear and at 0 dBHL in the 'deaf' ear. The level in the 'deaf' ear is raised in 5 dB steps. The patient should continue to respond because the tone that is 10 dB above threshold in the better ear will be readily

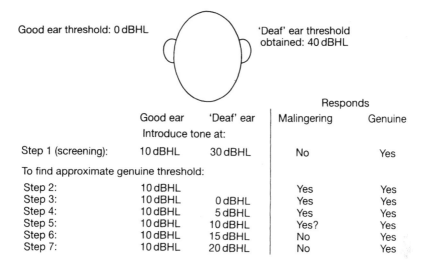

Good ear threshold: 0 dBHL

'Deaf' ear threshold obtained: 40 dBHL

	Good ear	'Deaf' ear	Responds Malingering	Genuine
	Introduce tone at:			
Step 1 (screening):	10 dBHL	30 dBHL	No	Yes
To find approximate genuine threshold:				
Step 2:	10 dBHL		Yes	Yes
Step 3:	10 dBHL	0 dBHL	Yes	Yes
Step 4:	10 dBHL	5 dBHL	Yes	Yes
Step 5:	10 dBHL	10 dBHL	Yes?	Yes
Step 6:	10 dBHL	15 dBHL	No	Yes
Step 7:	10 dBHL	20 dBHL	No	Yes

Fig. 12.9 The Stenger test procedure, used to determine whether an apparent hearing loss of 40 dBHL is true or non-organic.

heard (Figure 12.9). When the patient ceases to respond, the level in the 'deaf' ear is usually within 10 dB of its true threshold.

12.4.4 SUMMARY

Non-organic hearing loss is one that is not of organic origin. It may be feigned or exaggerated, often for financial gain, but it may also be of psychological origin. Non-organic hearing loss should be suspected whenever results of the different parts of the hearing assessment are at variance. The audiologist has to determine whether a hearing loss exists, and the true thresholds. A number of tests are available for suspected cases of non-organic hearing loss, for example the Lombard test and the delayed speech feedback test, which are based on interfering with normal auditory monitoring. The most widely used test for unilateral non-organic hearing losses is the Stenger test, which is based on the principle that it is only possible to hear the most intense of two tones of the same frequency presented simultaneously. Most tests set out to confuse the patient in order to provide evidence of non-organic hearing loss. Some tests also indicate the approximate hearing threshold.

REFERENCE FOR SECTION 12.4

Brooks, D.N. and Geoghegan, P.M. (1992) Non-organic Hearing Loss in Young Persons: Transient Episode or Indicator of Deep-seated Difficulty. *British Journal of Audiology*, **26**(6), 347–50.

FURTHER READING FOR SECTION 12.4

Arlinger, S. (1989) *Manual of Practical Audiometry*, Volume I, Whurr Publishers, London.

Northern, J.L. and Downs, M.P. (1984) *Hearing in Children*, 3rd edn, Williams & Wilkins, Baltimore.

12.5 AUTOMATIC AUDIOMETRY

12.5.1 INDUSTRIAL SCREENING

Automatic audiometry allows the person under test to plot his or her own audiogram. The audiometer presents a tone that gradually increases in intensity. The patient presses a button as soon as the tone is heard and keeps it pressed for as long as the tone is heard. On pressing the button, the tone becomes fainter. As soon as the tone is inaudible, the patient releases the button. When the button is released, the intensity increases.

The level of the tone is automatically traced on an audiogram, either as the frequency gradually changes, or at certain fixed frequencies. The resultant zigzag line indicates the swing-width, which is the difference between audibility and inaudibility. The threshold of hearing is taken as the mid-point between the extremes at each frequency and this produces thresholds that are almost identical to those obtained with manual audiometry. The width of the tracing is, on average, 6–10 dB, but can vary. In extreme cases it may be as little as 3 dB or as much as 20 dB. Extremely narrow tracing widths were, at one time, thought to be related to the difference limen for intensity and so, indirectly, to recruitment. Most authorities now consider that the width of the tracing is really an indication of threshold doubt and certainty, although it may be suggestive of a cochlear lesion.

12.5.2 BÉKÈSY AUDIOMETRY

Békèsy audiometry goes beyond automatic recording of audiograms and can provide diagnostic information, although it is not widely used. The audiometer presents tones that may be continuous (C) or interrupted (I), typically with 2.5 interruptions per second. The interrupted tracing obtained approximates to the pure-tone threshold. Clinical interpretation involves comparison of the continuous with the interrupted tone. Jerger (1960) classified the types of audiogram that may be obtained (Figure 12.10). These are as follows.

Type I A type I audiogram is where the continuous and interrupted tracings overlap. In this case the threshold remains the same whether the tone is present continuously or pulsing on and

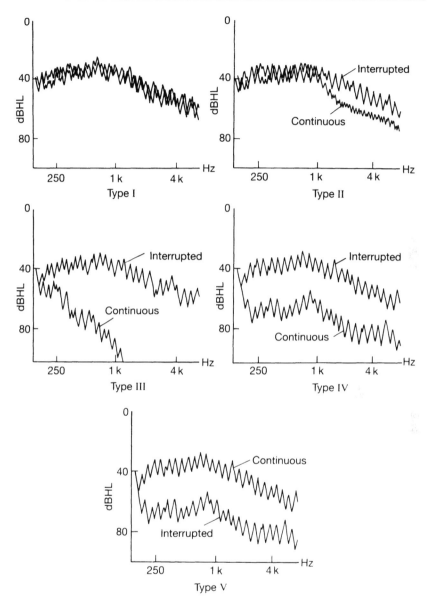

Fig. 12.10 Békèsy audiogram types, classified by Jerger (1960).

off. Type I tracings are obtained in patients with normal ears or with middle ear disorders.

Type II   A type II audiogram shows the continuous and interrupted tracings often overlapping in the low frequencies. From approximately 1 kHz the continuous tone appears to be more difficult to hear and the continuous trace drops below the interrupted trace. The continuous trace is rarely more than

20 dB below the interrupted trace, but the swing width may narrow. Type II audiograms are found mainly in patients with cochlear disorders.

Type III   At all frequencies the continuous tone falls dramatically below the interrupted tone. The patient appears to have marked adaptation and to find a continuous signal extremely difficult to hear. Type III audiograms are often found in patients with eighth nerve disorders.

Type IV   These audiograms are similar to type II except that the continuous tracing breaks away in the low frequency. These also tend to be obtained with eighth nerve disorders.

Type V   An audiogram in which the continuous tracing occurs above the interrupted tracing. This indicates a non-organic hearing loss.

The Békèsy audiogram types provide useful clinical information but are not sufficiently precise for diagnosis unless supported by other test results. In clinical practice, the frequency at which separation occurs tends to be ignored. No separation points to a conductive disorder, type II with a separation of up to 20 dB suggests a cochlear lesion, whereas an audiogram (excluding type V) with a separation of over 25 dB suggests a retrocochlear problem.

12.5.3 SUMMARY

Automatic audiometry allows patients to track their own pure-tone thresholds by pressing a button when the tone is audible and releasing the button when it is not. A pen tracks the resulting audiogram as a series of zigzag lines on a special audiogram form. Automatic audiometers are often used in industrial hearing conservation programmes. Clinical Békèsy audiometry provides diagnostic information through the comparison of the patient's response to continuous and to pulsed or interrupted tones. Five different audiogram types may be observed. These help in the differentiation of cochlear, retrocochlear and non-organic hearing losses.

REFERENCES FOR SECTION 12.5

Jerger, J. (1960) Hearing Tests in Otologic Diagnosis. *American Speech and Hearing Association*, **4**, 139–45.

FURTHER READING FOR SECTION 12.5

Arlinger, S. (1991) *Manual of Practical Audiometry*, Volume II, Whurr Publishers, London.

Paediatric provision 13

13.1 THE EFFECT OF HEARING LOSS IN CHILDREN

13.1.1 INTRODUCTION

Language forms the basis of our communication and our education. We all use language to adjust to our world. Without language our experience would be very different and our lives would be very difficult. Children begin to learn language skills from the very earliest age and their ability to understand and to use speech develops naturally over a very short space of time. The normal baby progresses from babble to using complex sentences in a period of less than three years. However, this rapid natural development is interrupted if a child cannot hear normally.

The age at which a hearing loss occurs is a critical factor in determining its effect on language development. Where a hearing loss occurs before the child has acquired speech it is termed 'prelingual'. Prelingual therefore covers a range of cases from those who were born deaf, to those who became deaf through illness, accident or other cause at an early stage – before about two years old. The term 'postlingual' is used where the child becomes deaf after learning to speak. Deafness from birth or acquired early in life has a serious effect on speech and language. The effect of a postlingual hearing loss on speech and language development is less serious, but in terms of education and social development may still be very traumatic.

In general terms, hearing loss acquired in childhood may affect:

- the development of speech and language;
- the ability to think abstractly;
- learning;
- social integration;
- social and emotional adjustment.

Speech difficulties are often seen as the primary problem for hearing impaired children, but they are really a reflection of the more central problem of poor comprehension. Even with early diagnosis and appropriate remediation, hearing impaired children's progress may be very delayed. Their inability to understand explanations, or to express their needs and feelings, may lead to frustration and socially unacceptable behaviour. There is an understandable tendency for parents to be over-protective, and normally-hearing siblings may become jealous of the time and money they feel is being diverted away from them.

The term 'hearing impaired' children includes all degrees of hearing loss from profound to very mild. As one would expect, the effects of such differing degrees of hearing loss may vary from marked to very slight. Many profoundly deaf children, for instance, fail to reach a reading level equivalent to that of an average eight-year-old by school leaving age (Conrad, 1977); the handicap of mild hearing loss is much less obvious.

Approximately 4 in every 1000 children have a significant sensorineural hearing loss (Haggard and Pullan, 1989).

13.1.2 TEMPORARY CONDUCTIVE HEARING LOSS

The most common cause of hearing loss in children is a temporary condition known as secretory or serous otitis media. It is so common that most children are affected by it at some stage in their early years (British Association of Audiological Physicians, 1990). It is a self-limiting condition and one out of which most children have grown by about eight years old. The problem is caused by fluid in the middle ear, which prevents the efficient passage of sound from the eardrum. In normality, the middle ear cavity is air-filled and it remains so because it is ventilated by the Eustachian tube. This tube runs from the middle ear to the back of the throat. In infants the Eustachian tubes are shorter, smaller and narrower than in adults, and they are positioned more horizontally. Ventilation and drainage of the ear of a child is therefore less efficient. If the Eustachian tube becomes blocked, air cannot enter the middle ear. Air is gradually absorbed by the lining of the middle ear cavity and cannot be replaced. The result is negative pressure in the middle ear and a thin watery fluid is secreted into the cavity. If the condition is not resolved the fluid may thicken and eventually become glue-like, hence the name 'glue ear', which is sometimes given to the disorder. Blockage of the Eustachian tube may be caused by a number of factors, including upper respiratory tract infections, enlarged tonsils and adenoids, allergies and malformations. The resulting hearing loss often fluctuates dramatically between a mild and a marked impairment. It is usually bilateral and rarely more than

60 dBHL in degree. In general, temporary fluctuating losses create more difficulty in the noisy conditions of school than they do in the less adverse conditions of the home where speech can be clear and close to the child. Minor conductive losses may not require medical intervention but will usually be monitored. Tympanometry can provide a simple check of middle ear function, and if treatment is required this will usually be medical or educational. Where speech and language are delayed, a child may also be referred to a speech and language therapist. Hearing aids should only be fitted if medical advice has been sought.

13.1.3 ASSESSMENT AND DIAGNOSIS OF HEARING LOSS IN CHILDREN

Pure-tone audiometry is not appropriate for very young children, and different diagnostic tests may be used depending on the age and mental ability of the child. The principle tests in use are:

1. brain stem evoked response (BSER);
2. distraction tests;
3. co-operative tests;
4. performance tests;
5. free-field visual response audiometry (VRA);
6. pure-tone audiometry.

Where ages are quoted these are only intended to provide a guide to the child's approximate stage of development.

(a) Brain stem evoked response audiometry

Brain Stem Evoked Response (BSER) is one type of evoked response audiometry (ERA) that can be used with young babies and other patients who are particularly difficult to test. Electrical potentials from the auditory pathways, in response to sounds, are recorded by electrodes attached to the baby's head. All levels of the sensorineural part of the auditory system, from the hair cells in the cochlea to the cortex of the brain, respond electrically to sound. The auditory responses are processed by a computer and displayed as a multiwave form. Changes in electrical potentials due to auditory activity are so small that they must be 'averaged' over a period of time in order that they can be singled out from the random activity of the brain.

ERA provides valuable objective results for a population that could not provide this information in any other way. BSER is the most widely used ERA for children. It may also be used in some cases of suspected non-organic hearing loss since no co-operation is required. It provides a good estimate of threshold, especially in the 2 kHz to 4 kHz region, and should be interpreted in the context of other clinical information.

(b) Distraction tests

Distraction tests are used both as a screening and a diagnostic test. They are suited to children between the ages of approximately 6 to 18 months, that is from the time the baby can sit unsupported and turn its head towards a sound, until it ceases to be sufficiently interested in the sounds to continue to turn reliably.

Two testers work as a team, one positioned at the front to attract and manipulate the child's attention, the other stands behind the child and presents the sound signals (Figure 13.1).

The object of the test is to record the quietest intensity at which the baby responds to a range of frequency-specific sounds. The sounds must be interesting to the baby and representative of low, mid- and high frequency ranges. Examples of those in common use include:

- low frequency – the voiced sound 'oo-oo' (approximately 500 Hz);
- midfrequency – a G-chime bar (approximately 1600 Hz);
- high frequency – a special high frequency rattle (above approximately 6.5 kHz) (Kettlety, 1987).

Responses must be obtained at 30 dB to pass a screening test, but in the diagnostic situation the intensity is raised until a response is obtained. The intensity is measured using a sound level meter.

It is extremely important to be certain that the child is really responding to the auditory signal and not to other clues. Some children are very quick to respond to the touch of the tester's breath, the sound of a footfall, the smell of perfume or the movement of a shadow. These are known, respectively, as tactile, auditory, olfactory or visual

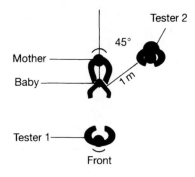

Fig. 13.1 The position of two testers carrying out a distraction test. The baby is sat upright on the mother's knee. Tester 1 manipulates the baby's attention, while tester 2 presents the sound signals.

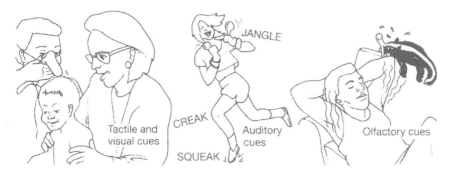

Fig. 13.2 A tester may obtain false positive responses during a distraction test if other cues are present; such cues may be auditory, visual, tactile or olfactory. (After Anon.)

cues (Figure 13.2). Distraction tests appear very simple to the observer but they must be meticulously performed to be reliable.

(c) Co-operative tests

Co-operative tests are used for children aged between about 18 months and two and a half years, when the baby has become too 'grown up' to respond reliably to distraction techniques but is not yet able to perform the next level of test. This age group is, contrary to the name of the test, notoriously uncooperative. One tester is needed to carry out this simple speech test, which provides only limited low frequency information and is therefore used in conjunction with a brief high frequency distraction test.

The child is supplied with bricks or similar toys and the tester gives simple instructions. There is a limited choice of instruction, such as 'Give it to Mummy', 'Give it to Daddy', 'Give it to teddy', and the lowest intensity at which the child can respond accurately is found. A child with normal hearing should be able to achieve this at a level of 40–45 dBA.

(d) Performance tests

Performance tests can be useful from the age of about two and a half, until the child is able to undertake pure-tone audiometry. The child is trained or 'conditioned' to perform an action, such as placing a man in a boat, whenever he or she hears a 'command' sound, which for low frequencies is 'go', and for high frequencies is the sibilant 's'. The intensity of the command is gradually reduced until the child's hearing threshold is obtained. The intensity is measured, as in all free-field tests, using a sound level meter.

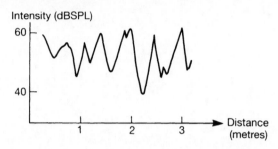

Fig. 13.3 Intensity variation of a pure-tone due to standing waves.

(e) Visual response audiometry

Visual response audiometry, often known as 'VRA', is a technique that requires more complex equipment than distraction tests but that can be used for the whole age range, from about six months until the child can perform pure-tone audiometry.

Loudspeakers are used to deliver frequency-specific signals, in the form of warble tones or narrow band noise. A warble tone is a sound that continually changes in frequency around a centre frequency. A 1 kHz warble tone could, for example, have a band width of 10% and vary between 950 Hz and 1050 Hz. Warble tones and narrow band noise are used in place of pure tones to avoid standing waves. If pure tones were used in the test room, reflections would cause interference with the intensity of the signal, creating standing waves (Figure 13.3).

Young children do not find electronically-produced tones very interesting and some form of visual reinforcement is therefore used, often in the form of a toy that lights up when the child responds correctly. Since headphones are not worn, the information obtained will relate to the better ear and, when high intensities are used, the signal can be distorted and no longer frequency specific. Nevertheless, a limited audiogram may be obtained in this way, usually providing points at 500 Hz, 1 kHz, (2 kHz) and 4 kHz.

(f) Pure-tone audiometry

Pure-tone audiometry should be used as soon as the child is able to co-operate reliably since the ears can be tested separately. Many children from around the age of three can be trained to carry out a pure-tone test if it is treated as a game. 'Play techniques' are used in which the child is taught to respond to the tones by performing some action, such as placing a peg in a board.

A restricted range of frequencies is often tested, such as 500 Hz, 1 kHz and 4 kHz, since the child may lose concentration before a full test can be completed. Masking is also usually possible with children from about five years old, if the instructions are simplified and the 'play-like' nature of the test is retained.

13.2 HABILITATION OF HEARING IMPAIRED CHILDREN

13.2.1 THE HABILITATION PROCESS

A multidisciplinary team is usually involved with the diagnosis and management of the hearing impaired child. Such a team may include:

- audiological physician or otologist;
- clinical or educational audiologist;
- teacher of the deaf;
- educational psychologist;
- social worker;
- other specialists.

In the initial stages parents have to come to terms with the child's impairment, and it is usually the audiological physician or otologist who counsels the parents and who will answer any medical questions they may have. Parents may feel a sense of guilt, numbness, fear and isolation, feelings with which they have to come to terms before they can help their child. After the initial diagnosis, support and counselling will be undertaken by a peripatetic teacher of the deaf, who will see the family on a regular basis, in the home and, later, in the school.

The selection of appropriate hearing aids is central to the rehabilitation process in order to provide maximum use of residual hearing. The fundamental principles of hearing aid selection are the same for children as for adults, but provision should be made as early as possible, with binaural fitting considered as the norm. It is also important that hearing aids are worn constantly from the beginning, and that they are checked regularly by an adult to ensure they are working.

Hearing aids for children usually need repairing at least once a year and replacing every three to four years (British Association of Audiological Physicians, 1990). In addition, new earmoulds are required several times a year and batteries need frequent replacement.

There are three main types of personal hearing aid systems in use with hearing impaired children at present: bodyworn, postaural and in-the-ear aids. The most widely used system is currently the postaural hearing aid. In-the-ear hearing aids are increasing in popularity but these have to be replaced or re-shelled at frequent intervals as the child grows.

Where audiological and other factors allow for choice of the hearing aid system, parental feelings should be taken into consideration. If the parents of the child are not happy with the hearing aid system, the child is unlikely to make the best use of it. Many children are provided with commercial hearing aids under the National Health Service when it is felt there is a need that cannot be met by the standard range. The reasons for this are varied but may include requirements for:

- mini-postaural hearing aids for small ears;
- compression or automatic gain control;
- difficult audiometric configurations that cannot be adequately fitted with the standard range of frequency response;
- direct input facility for radio hearing aids used mainly in education.

Many children, particularly those with severe and profound losses, are provided with radio hearing aids in addition to their personal aids. These overcome some of the problems of interference from background noise.

13.2.2 RADIO HEARING AID SYSTEMS

Personal hearing aids depend for their effectiveness on being used close to the speaker, in order to achieve a high 'signal-to-noise' ratio. When the speaker moves away the increasing distance quickly results in a weak signal that is lost in the masking effect of background noise.

In schools, background noise and reverberation are often such as to reduce the effectiveness of hearing aids significantly (Figure 13.4).

Radio frequency modulated (FM) systems are used to provide a short microphone distance. The microphone is worn by the teacher and the pupil wears a radio receiver, which is linked to a hearing aid. The

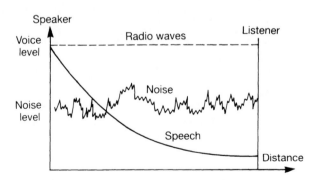

Fig. 13.4 As the distance away from the speaker increases, the intensity of the signal falls (according to the inverse square law). Background noise then interferes with the speech signal received by the hearing aid.

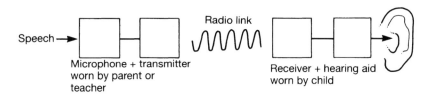

Fig. 13.5 The basic format of a radio hearing aid.

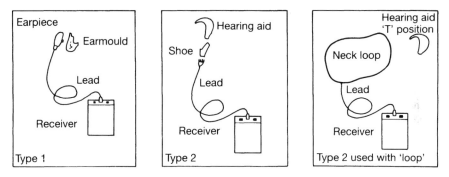

Fig. 13.6 The child's unit in each of the types of radio system.

signal is transmitted to the pupil, regardless of his or her position, up to a distance of about 100 metres from the microphone (Figure 13.5). Radio hearing aids are used at school and at home, and to a limited extent by adults, but their use is restricted by their expense and their appearance, which is similar to a large bodyworn aid.

There are two types of radio systems (Figure 13.6).

Type 1 is a complete radio hearing aid, in which the radio receiver is also a bodyworn hearing aid. These tend to by used by some profoundly deaf children, although they could equally well be used for children with mild hearing losses who do not otherwise use a hearing aid. The main reason for not doing so is the expense, as radio hearing aids are very costly.

Type 2 is a system used in conjunction with the child's individual hearing aid. This is the type most widely used because it provides continuation of hearing through the same hearing aid. The radio receiver is usually linked directly into the personal hearing aid via a lead and shoe; this is known as 'direct input'. In some cases the system is used with a neck loop which permits the whole receiving unit to be hidden under clothing, but the performance of the induction loop tends to be inferior to that of direct input due to a reduced low frequency response and an increased tendency to interference, mainly from fluorescent lights and other electrical sources.

13.2.3 EDUCATIONAL PROVISION

Many hearing impaired children will need educational support from the time of diagnosis throughout their education. Most hearing impaired children are educated within the ordinary, or 'mainstream', school system, with varying degrees of support. Ordinary schools provide an environment in which the child can gain experience of normal language and behaviour, benefit from a wide curriculum, make friends among local children and, in general, learn to adjust to being part of the hearing world.

For children with a significant hearing loss support is usually provided in the form of personal hearing aids, a radio system and the services of a peripatetic, or visiting, teacher of the deaf. However, ordinary schools tend to be large, noisy and often intolerant places and some children are unable to cope. Hearing impaired children may be placed in:

- normal 'mainstream' school;
- special class, or 'unit', within the ordinary school;
- special school.

Children who need significant extra support may be provided with a 'statement of educational needs', under the 1981 Education Act. A statement formalizes the child's special needs and ways of meeting these, while reinforcing the parent's right to be involved in the process.

A special class or 'partially hearing unit' is an attempt to provide 'the best of both worlds', with children integrated into ordinary classes as far as possible, but having an individual programme tailored to their needs, and with access to a full-time teacher of the deaf.

Special school provision has decreased, as children are increasingly placed within the normal school environment. Most of the special schools that do remain cater for the needs of particular groups of severely and profoundly deaf children, such as those who are:

- in need of a high level of support;
- of a particular religion;
- academically very able;
- using an alternative method of communication;
- multiply handicapped.

Children in special schools have less access to 'normal' patterns of speech and of behaviour and may be less prepared for coping with the demands of everyday life, but special schools can provide a con-

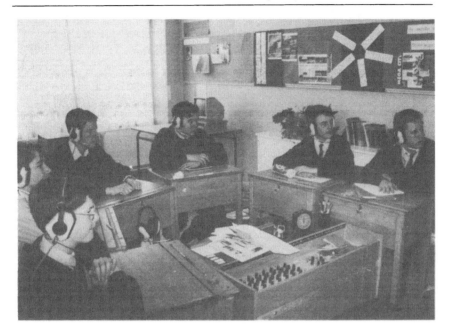

Fig. 13.7 A group hearing aid system, in use at St John's School for Deaf Children, Boston Spa, West Yorkshire.

centration of specialist staff and facilities. Children are educated within a protected environment and in very small classes, consisting of not more than ten children. Classrooms can be sound-treated, and specialist equipment often includes group hearing aids and speech training units. A group hearing aid is a hard-wire system in which each child wears headphones linked to a desk unit capable of providing high output over an extended frequency range and, since the ear is not blocked, advantage is also taken of ear canal resonance. The teacher uses a microphone that is also wired into the system (Figure 13.7). Speech training equipment includes individual hard-wire hearing aid units, often with a visual display to help the child monitor his or her speech.

Approaches to the education of very severely and profoundly deaf children vary markedly, especially between an 'oral' or 'manual' approach. All systems make use of hearing aids and strive to develop language and learning. Unfortunately, deep divisions exist between the supporters of the various approaches, which is often unhelpful to parents since they receive conflicting advice. Most hearing impaired children can learn to communicate by speech if their loss is diagnosed early and treated promptly with effective hearing aids and skilled guidance. In essence, 'oral' methods seek to develop speech in a natural manner, while manual or 'total' communication provides support to the spoken pattern in one of a number of ways, namely using:

- sign language – this is often said to be the natural language of the deaf community, although unfortunately there is no one universally recognized sign language and few hearing people are able to sign, except in a slow and clumsy manner;
- finger-spelling – this can be likened to the written pattern and is of limited use until the child has achieved some proficiency in language;
- cued speech – this is a method of communication in which hand positions are used to supplement the information available through lip-reading.

Special consideration must be given to the education of hearing impaired children. Hearing loss provides a starting point but is not a sufficient basis on which to make a decision. The child's whole development and his or her family's wishes should be considered in selecting an appropriate school placement.

13.3 SUMMARY

Hearing impairment in childhood hinders development of the ability to communicate and to make normal progress in school. Early diagnosis and appropriate management are among the factors that can reduce the handicapping effect of hearing loss. Evaluation of hearing in early childhood necessitates the use of special techniques appropriate to a child's age and stage of development. Educational placement should take full account of the child's needs and the parents' wishes. Great emphasis is placed on the full use of residual hearing through amplification in all educational environments, and support is provided by specialist teachers of the deaf. Most hearing impaired children are able to receive their education with the normally-hearing in 'mainstream' school, with the necessary specialist support.

REFERENCES

Conrad, R. (1977) The Reading Ability of Deaf School Leavers. *British Journal of Educational Psychology*, **47**, 138–48.

British Association of Audiological Physicians (1990) *Paediatric Audiological Medicine – Into the 1990s, Policy Document*, The British Association of Audiological Physicians.

Haggard, M.P. and Pullan, C.R. (1989) The Staffing and Structure for Paediatric Audiology Services in Hospital and Community Units. *British Journal of Audiology*, **23**(2), 99–116.

Kettlety, A. (1987) The Manchester High Pitch Rattle. *British Journal of Audiology*, **21**, 73–4.

FURTHER READING

Davies, H. and Fallowfield, L. (1991) *Counselling and Communication in Health Care*, J. Wiley and Sons, Chichester.

McCormick, B. (1988) *Paediatric Audiology 0–5 years*, Taylor and Francis, London.

Murgatroyd, S. (1985) *Counselling and Helping*, Methuen, London.

National Deaf Children's Society (1990) *Audiological Services for Children – Recommended Practice*, The National Deaf Children's Society, London.

Nolan, M. and Tucker, I. (1988) *The Hearing Impaired Child and the Family*, Souvenir Press, London.

Northern, J.L. and Downs, M.P. (1984) *Hearing in Children*, 3rd edn, Williams and Wilkins, Baltimore.

Tucker, I. and Nolan, M. (1984) *Educational Audiology*, Croom Helm, London.

Appendix   Glossary

TERM	MEANING
A-Scale	The weighting network used with a sound level meter for free-field sound measurements. The A-Scale approximates to the inverted 40 phon equal loudness curve.
Acoustic feedback	The excitation of the microphone by sound generated from the receiver of the same system.
Acoustic neuroma	Benign eighth nerve tumour.
Acoustic ohm	Unit of acoustic impedance.
Acoustic reflex	Contraction of middle ear muscles in response to loud sound.
Acoustic trauma	Noise damage due to sudden impulse noise of high intensity.
Acoustics	Study of science of sound.
Action potential	Brief electrical discharge which occurs when a cell is activated.
Acute	Short and severe.
Adaptation	Reduction in hearing sensitivity within a brief time of the sound onset.
Adhesion	New and abnormal tissue growth due to inflammation.
Admittance	The ease with which sound waves pass through.
Air–bone gap	The difference in dB between the air conduction reading on an audiogram and the bone conduction reading for the same ear. If greater than 10 dB indicates a conductive element.
Alport's syndrome	Kidney disorder combined with hearing and sight defects.

Ambient	Surrounding or background.
Amplitude	The maximum displacement of any wave from its equilibrium position.
Analgesic	Pain-killing drug, e.g. aspirin.
Anechoic	With no echoes or significant sound reflection: 'dead'.
Anoxia	Lack of oxygen.
Aphasia	Disorder of central nervous system causing difficulty with speech and language.
Artificial ear	A 6cc coupling device used in audiometer earphone calibration.
Artificial mastoid	Calibration device for bone vibrators, which simulates the mechanical impedance of an average normal human mastoid.
Atresia	Absence of an opening.
Attenuation	Reduction.
Audiogram	A graph showing a person's hearing thresholds for pure-tones.
Audiometry	The measurement of hearing.
Auditory adaptation	Decrease in hearing sensitivity within a brief time of the sound onset.
Auditory training	Teaching a hearing impaired person to make best use of residual hearing.
Aural	Of the ear.
Aural–oral approach	A method of teaching hearing impaired children using speech and hearing optimally.
Auricle	Pinna.
Auropalpebral reflex (APR)	Eye-blink in response to loud sound.
Automatic gain control (AGC)	Automatic reduction in gain of a hearing aid to avoid user discomfort and with minimum distortion of the sound signal.
Azimuth	Distance in degrees, e.g. 0° azimuth = straight ahead; 90° azimuth = to person's right.
Barotrauma	Injury to ear due to sudden pressure change.
Behavioural audiometry	Assessment of hearing by noting bodily responses.
Békèsy audiometry	Automatic audiometry.
Benign	Not of cancer.
Binaural summation	Improvement in hearing threshold when hearing via both ears. Usually at least 3dB and may be much more.
Brief tone	Tone of 500 milliseconds or less.

Calibration	Checking, and adjusting if necessary, the output of a measurement device, e.g. audiometer.
Central	In brain and/or spinal cord.
Cholesteatoma	Cyst-like growth in the middle ear containing shed skin.
Chronic	Having lasted a long time.
Click	A short impulse of sound, too short in duration for its characteristics to be fully perceived.
CMV	Cytomegalovirus disease.
Cochlear microphonic	Electrical output from cochlear hair cells, following input signal.
Compliance	Opposite of stiffness; ability to give.
Compression	Limiting of maximum output, using automatic gain control.
Conditioning	Rewarding of required behaviour, used widely in assessment of children.
Congenital	Present at birth.
Contralateral	On the opposite side.
Critical band	The narrow band of noise required to mask a pure-tone signal.
Cross-hearing	Sound presented to one ear is perceived in the other by vibration of the skull.
Derecruitment	Abnormally slow growth of loudness, usually due to disorder of auditory nerve.
Dichotic	Affecting each ear differently.
Difference limen (e.g. of intensity or frequency)	The smallest detectable difference between two signals.
Digital hearing aid	The electrical signal is converted to digital values for modification before being converted back to an electrical signal which is passed to the receiver.
Diotic	Identical signal to each ear.
Diplacusis	One pure-tone appears to the listener as two or more tones.
Directional microphone	One that is more responsive to sound from one direction – normally the front.
Distortion	Any unwanted sound present in the output that was not present in the input.
Diuretic	Drug to increase urination.
Down's syndrome	A congenital abnormality, formerly known as mongolism. Features include mental retar-

	dation, Mongoloid eyes, flattened facial features, short, broad hands and feet, small pinnae, narrow ear canals and a high incidence of conductive and sensorineural hearing loss.
Dynamic range	The difference in dB between the threshold of hearing and the threshold of discomfort.
Earhook	That part of a postaural aid that fits over the ear. The elbow.
Earphone	A loudspeaker at the ear.
Ear simulator	A coupler that simulates the acoustic characteristics of an average adult ear.
Effective gain	The difference between aided and unaided thresholds.
Effusion	An abnormal outpouring of fluid.
Electro-acoustic device	A device that converts electrical to acoustic signals and vice versa.
Electrocochleography	Recording electrical signals (action potentials) from the eighth nerve.
Environmental microphone	A microphone that picks up airborne sound – for example, an environmental microphone may be built into a radio hearing aid so the pupils can hear themselves and their colleagues as well as the teacher.
Fall time	The time needed for a signal to decay by 60 dB from its steady state.
Feedback (acoustic)	The whistling that occurs from a hearing aid when sound leaks from the receiver and is picked up and re-amplified via the microphone.
Feedback	Information that is used to maintain or modify performance.
Filter (acoustic)	Allows some sounds to pass but attenuates others.
Formant	A special pattern of speech sounds, determined by the vocal cords and the resonant cavities of the vocal tract, giving each vowel its recognizable quality.
Fossa	Groove.
Free-field	Open space – or an area with boundaries that are negligible for the test.
Frequency analyser	A sound level meter with an octave band (or

	other) filter. Displays amplitude versus frequency on graph of input.
Functional gain	Real ear gain.
Functional hearing loss	Non-organic or psychogenic.
Fundamental	The lowest frequency in a periodic waveform.
Harmonic	A frequency that is a whole number multiple of the pure-tone to which it is related.
Haematoma	Blood clot due to a break in a blood vessel.
Hertz	A unit used in the measurement of frequency of sound, equivalent to the number of cycles per second.
High-pass filter	Reduces low frequencies while allowing high frequencies to pass unaffected.
Homeostasis	Equilibrium – achieving a normal balance.
Horn	A tapered sound tube.
Hypacusis	Loss of hearing.
Idiopathic	Cause unknown.
Immitance	Impedance or admittance.
Impedance (acoustic)	Resistance to the passage of sound.
Impedance match	Making the resistance of two connecting parts equal.
Incidence	The number of cases in a given population (e.g. as a number of live births).
Incident wave	Any wave that has its path interrupted by an object; the wave is then said to be incident on this object.
Induction coil	Picks up electromagnetic signals from a loop amplifier; activated in a hearing aid by the 'T' switch.
Inflammation	Sore, swollen, red area.
Insertion gain	The difference between the gain of the open ear and the gain of the ear wearing a hearing aid, i.e. aided − unaided real ear gain.
Insertion loss	The difference between the gain of the open ear and that of an occluded ear.
In situ	In the natural position.
Intelligibility	The understanding of speech.
Interaural attenuation	The degree to which sound is reduced as it crosses the head. Minimum interaural attenuation is 40 dB for air conducted signals and 0 dB for bone conduction.

Intermodulation	Frequencies in the output that are the sum and the difference of two or more input frequencies and their harmonics.
Intonation	Pitch variation.
Ipsilateral	On the same side.
Isthmus	A narrowed part of an organ or tissue.
Labyrinthitis	Inflammation of the labyrinth.
Latency	The time delay between a stimulus and the response to that stimulus.
Lateralization	When sound appears to be heard on one side although the signal was placed on the other side or in the centre of the head (as in certain tuning fork tests).
Lesion	An injury.
Lexicon	Vocabulary.
Linear	A straight line, this applies when a change of input causes the same change in output.
Localization	Ability to pin-point a sound source.
Loop (amplifier)	An amplifying system which uses electromagnetic induction. A loop of wire is placed around the room and a current is induced in a coil within the hearing aid. Helps to overcome interference from background noise.
Loudspeaker	Apparatus that converts electrical impulses into sound.
Low-pass filter	Allows low frequency sound to pass, but attenuates high frequencies.
Mainstream	Education within a normal school.
Malignant	Cancerous, may cause death.
Mandibulofacial dysplasia	Treacher Collin's syndrome.
Manometer	An instrument to measure pressure.
Manual audiometry	As carried out by the hearing aid dispenser or audiologist by the normal methods.
Masker	An instrument used in the management of tinnitus; produces a continuous masking noise.
Masking	Raising of the threshold of hearing for one sound by the introduction of another.
Maximum power output	Saturation or output sound pressure level. The greatest amount of sound pressure or intensity the hearing aid can produce under any circumstances.

Menière's disorder	Idiopathic episodic endolymphatic hydrops. A syndrome or disorder in which there is fluctuating sensorineural hearing loss, vertigo and tinnitus, due to excessive fluid pressure in the inner ear.
Meningitis	Inflammation of the brain lining.
Mixed loss	A hearing loss that is a combination of conductive and sensorineural type.
Monaural	One ear.
Monitored	Regulated – often of live voice using a sound level meter.
Myringoplasty	Surgery to repair a perforated tympanic membrane.
Myringotomy	Surgical incision of tympanic membrane.
Narrow band	A small range of frequencies.
Neck loop	A small loop of wire worn around the user's neck, rather than having a loop placed around the room (see 'Loop').
Neoplasm	A new tumour.
Neuroma	A tumour.
Noise	i) Unwanted sound or unwanted electrical signal. ii) Aperiodic or non-periodic sound.
Non-invasive	Not involving surgery.
Non-organic	Not of physical origin, as in psychological or fake.
Null	Negative (as in a negative response) or void.
Nystagmus	Involuntary beating movements of the eyes.
Objective	Able to be observed or measured; not subjective.
Occluded	Closed.
Occlusion effect	An apparent improvement in hearing by bone conduction when the external auditory meatus is occluded.
Omnidirectional microphone	Accepts sound equally from all directions.
On-effect	The greatest response, which occurs at the onset of a signal.
Oscillator	A sound source.
Osteogenesis imperfecta	Brittle bones.
Otalgia	Earache.

Otitis	Inflammation of the ear.
Otitis media	Inflammation of the middle ear.
Otolaryngology	Ear, nose and throat (ENT) medical specialty.
Otology	Ear medical specialty.
Otorrhoea	Discharge from the ear.
Otosclerosis	Bone growth disorder affecting stapes and causing conductive hearing loss.
Ototoxic	Potentially poisonous to the ear.
Over-masking	Too much masking, which may affect the test ear and worsen its threshold.
Overshoot	An initial level reached which is greater than the steady state of a signal.
Paget's disease	Thickening and softening of bones, especially of skull.
Palsy	Paralysis.
Paracusis	Abnormal hearing (see Willis' paracusis).
Parameter	A variable or attribute.
Pascal	Unit of pressure equivalent to 1 newton per square metre.
Perinatal	Around the time of birth.
Peripheral	Not within the central nervous system.
Phase	Part of the period of a sound wave – can be expressed in degrees.
Phon	A unit of equal loudness.
Phoneme	The smallest individual speech sound.
Phonetic balance	Having the same distribution of speech sounds as a random sample of everyday conversational English.
Pip	A pure-tone with a rapid rise time and having a steady state that is no more than one cycle in length.
Polarity	Positive or negative (as in electricity).
Pontine	In that part of the brain stem known as the pons.
Postauricular	Behind the ear.
Postlingual	After the acquisition of speech.
Potentiometer	Variable control in a hearing aid.
Prelingual	Before the acquisition of speech.
Presbyacusis	Loss of hearing with old age.
Probe (tube) microphone	Used in real ear measurements to measure sound from near the tympanic membrane.
Prosthesis	An artificial replacement for an impaired body part.

Pseudohypacusis	Non-organic or functional hearing loss.
Psychoacoustics	Concerned with the relationship between measured signals and their subjective attributes.
Quiescent current	Current in a transistor in the absence of a driving or input signal.
Receiver	A term coined by the hearing aid industry to mean loudspeaker.
Recruitment	Abnormal loudness growth, usually found with cochlear impairment.
Redundancy	Part of the speech message that can be omitted without loss of meaning.
Rehabilitation	Therapy to help restore (normal) functioning.
Reliability	Consistency – how repeatable is a test.
Residual hearing	That part of the normal dynamic range that the impaired person is left with.
Resonance	Minimum acoustic impedance that occurs at a particular frequency, that is, a higher SPL will be recorded at this (resonant) frequency than at any other.
Retrocochlear	Beyond the cochlea.
Reverberation	Continuation of sound by reflecting or echoing.
Rise time	The time taken for a signal to reach its steady state.
Roll off	Rate of attenuation in dB per octave.
Room acoustics	How the design of a room affects the sound within it.
Rubella	German measles.
Saturation	Maximum – any further increase in input will cause no increase in output.
Sensation level	Amount above the individual's threshold.
Sensorineural	Impairment caused in or beyond the cochlea.
Sequelae	After effects of disease.
Sibilant	High frequency consonant of a hissing nature, e.g. 's' as in sue, 'ʃ' as in shoe.
Signal to noise ratio	Signal level compared to the competing noise. Usually expressed as signal minus noise, e.g. a signal of 60 dBA with a competing noise level of 50 dBA gives S:N of +10 dB.
Signs	Signs of a disorder are whatever features are noted by the doctor, e.g. swelling, discharge, redness.

Sintered mesh	A filter made of partially-fused metal.
Sound field	Containing sound waves, e.g. in a room.
Sound level meter	A device to measure sound pressure in dB.
Sound pressure level	SPL – a scale in which 0 dB = 20 micro Pascals.
Spectograph	A three-dimensional display of the energy of speech. Frequency and time are represented by the two axes of the graph. Intensity is shown by the darkness of the trace.
Speech spectrum	The average level of the speech sounds.
Speech reception threshold	The faintest level at which a person can identify 50% in a speech test.
Speech-reading	Lip-reading – but includes use of all cues not just those visible on the lips.
Spondee	A two-syllable word with equal stress on each syllable, e.g. football.
Stapedectomy	Removal of the stapes and replacement with a prosthesis.
Stenosis	Narrowing of the canal, as in stenosis of the external auditory meatus.
Submucous	Below the skin and surface tissue.
Supra-aural	On (against) the ear.
Suprasegmental	Features of speech that add to the phonemes, e.g. time, intonation, pitch, loudness.
Suprathreshold	Above threshold.
Sweep frequency	A tone that gradually changes across a frequency range.
Symptoms	Features that are complained of by a patient, e.g. pain, throbbing, heat, noises.
Syndrome	A group of features that characterize a disorder.
Telecoil	Induction coil in loop amplification system.
Temporal	Concerned with time.
Tinnitus	Noises in the ear or head with no external source.
Tolerance	Ability to hear sound without discomfort.
Tone burst	Tone with rapid rise time and short duration.
Tone decay	Decrease in hearing sensitivity when a tone is held for a short time, e.g. 1–3 minutes.
Transducer	A device to change one type of energy to another, e.g. sound energy to electricity.
Transient tone	A brief tone, of 500 milliseconds or less.
Trauma	Injury.
Trimmer	An adjustable element.
Tympanometry	Measurement of the ease or difficulty with which sound passes through the eardrum.

Unilateral	Of one side.
Unoccluded	Open.
Upward spread of masking	Low frequency sounds mask higher frequency sounds.
Validity	The degree to which a test measures what it was intended to measure.
Vent	A hole drilled through an ear mould, usually to release unwanted low frequency sounds.
Vertigo	Disturbance of balance.
Vibrotactile	Feeling vibration.
Viseme	Phonemes that appear the same to a lip-reader, e.g. 'p', 'b' and 'm'.
Warble tone	A frequency modulated tone; the tone varies around a central frequency. Used to avoid standing waves in free-field testing.
Wavelength	The distance covered in one cycle of a sound.
White noise	Broad band noise in which each frequency is presented at equal intensity.
Willis' paracusis	An apparent ability to hear better in the presence of background noise.
Zwislocki coupler	One particular model of occluded ear simulator. Simulates the acoustic impedance of the average adult ear.

Index

ABLB, *see* Alternate binaural loudness balance test
AB word list 192–3
Acoustic filters 184–5
Acoustic impedance 233–4
Acoustic neuroma 57
Acoustic reflex 34, 235, 237–9
Acoustics 3–19
Acquired conditions of the ear 42–6, 47–50, 53–7
Adaptation 245
Addition cured silicone 174–5
Afferent nerve fibres 29–30
AGC, *see* Automatic gain control
Aided thresholds 190
Air–bone gap 118–20
Air conduction hearing aids 127–32
Air conduction output transducer (hearing aid) 82, 83
Air conduction threshold testing 106
Alternate binaural loudness balance test 241–4
American National Standards Institute 140, 141
Amplifiers
  class A 79, 87, 147
  class AB 79–81, 87, 147
  class B, *see* class AB
  class D 81–2
Anatomy 20–32
ANSI, *see* American National Standards Institute
Aperiodic sound 9
Artificial mastoid 145–6
'A' scale 12, 14, 18
ASP, *see* Automatic signal processing
Assistive devices 213–14

Atresia 42
Attack time 89, 138–9
Audiogram
  interpretation 118–20
  pure tone 117
  speech 196
  symbols 114, 117–18
Audiological assessment
  audiogram interpretation 118–21
  case history 97–8
  masking 109–16
  otoscopy 101–3
  pure tone audiometry 106–9
  referrable conditions 98–101
  tuning fork tests 103–5
Audiological reference pressure 11
Audiometer 14–17
  calibration 14–16
  configuration 15
  daily checks 16
  speech 195
  standards 15–16
Audiometric room requirements 122–3
Audiometric symbols 114, 117–18
Audiometric test frequencies 15, 107–8
Audiometric tests 106–8
Audiometry
  automatic 250–2
  impedance 232–9
  masking 109–16
  paediatric 255–9
  pure tone 106–9
  speech 191–7
Auditory adaptation 245
Auditory deprivation 159

Auditory feedback   71–2
Auditory pathways, *see* Central
    connections of cochlear nerve
Auditory training   212–13, 218
Auditory tube, *see* Eustachian tube
Aural rehabilitation, *see* Rehabilitation
Auricle, *see* Pinna
Automatic audiometry   250–2
Automatic gain control   88–91,
    138–9, 170–1
Automatic signal processing   92
Automatic volume control, *see*
    Automatic gain control
Auxiliary aids, *see* Assistive devices
Average speech spectrum   70, 164

Background noise reduction   92
    see also Bass cut; Venting
Bacterial conditions of the ear, *see*
    Infection
Balance, organ of   30
Basilar membrane   29, 35–6
Bass cut   86–7
    see also Automatic signal processing;
    Venting
Batteries, hearing aid   146–9
Battery life   147
Behind-the-ear hearing aid   128–9
Békèsy audiometry   250–2
Békèsy's travelling wave theory
    35–6
Bi-CROS hearing aids   162–3
Binaural hearing   157
    advantages over monaural   157–60
Bodyworn hearing aid   127–8
Bone conduction hearing aid   132
Bone conduction output transducer
    82, 83
Bone conduction threshold testing
    107–8
Bone vibrator, *see* Bone conduction
    output transducer
Bone vibrator output measurement
    145
Brain stem evoked response
    audiometry   255–6
British Standards Institution   140
BTE, *see* Behind-the-ear hearing aid

Canal hearing aid, *see* In-the-canal
    hearing aid
Carhart's notch   50, 108

Case history   97–8
Causes of hearing loss, *see* Medical
    aspects of hearing loss
Central connections of cochlear nerve
    38–9
Cholesteatoma   49
Cochlea   27–30
Cochlear fluids   27
Cochlear hearing loss, *see*
    Sensorineural hearing loss
Cochlear hearing loss, tests of   241–5
Cochlear innervation   29
Cochlear potentials   37–8
Code of practice   215–17
    referrable conditions   98–101
Complex sound   7
Compliance   235–7
Compression   89, 91
Condensation reaction silicone   174
Conductive hearing loss   42–50, 60,
    108, 118–19, 238, 254–5
Congenital conditions of the ear   42,
    46–7, 51–3
Consonants   67–8
Contralateral routeing of signals
    130, 161–3
Corti, organ of   28–9
Counselling, *see* Rehabilitation
Coupler, 2cc   143, 144, 166
Couplers   142–3
CROS hearing aid   130, 161–3
Cross hearing   108, 109–10
Crouzon's syndrome   46
Current, electrical   84–5
Cytomegalovirus (CMV)   53

dBHL, *see* Decibel, hearing level
dBSPL, *see* Decibel, sound pressure
    level
Decibel
    hearing level   12
    scales   7, 10–12
    sound pressure level   7
Delayed speech feedback test   248
Directional microphone   77–8
Disease, *see* Pathology
Discharge, ear   99
    see also Otitis externa; Otitis media
Distortion   136–8
Doerfler–Stewart test   248
Down's syndrome   46
Drugs, *see* Ototoxic drugs

Dynamic range of hearing   12, 13, 116

Ear
  anatomy   20–32
  canal, *see* External auditory meatus
  canal resonance   188
  physiology   32–40
  simulator   142–3
Earache   58–9, 99
Ear examination   175–6
  see also Otoscopy
Earmould
  materials   178–9
  types   179–81
Earmoulds   173, 174, 178–85
Ear impression   173
  equipment   175
  technique   176–8
Echo   10
Eczema   45
Educational audiology   262–4
Efferent nerve fibres   29–30
Electret microphone   77
Electrical conduction   84–5
Electricity, elementary theory   84–5
Electro-acoustic impedance   234–5
Endolymph   27
Equivalent input noise level   138
ERA, *see* Evoked response audiometry
Eustachian tube   24, 26, 47–9, 254
Evaluation of hearing aids   187–99
Evoked response audiometry   255–6
Excessive wax   44, 99, 176
External auditory meatus   20, 22, 33
  see also Otoscopy

Fall time   16–17
Feedback
  acoustic   209–10
  auditory   71–2
Filters, acoustic   184–5
Fluctuating hearing loss   100
Formants   66
Frequency
  audible range   5
  fundamental   8
  of sound   5–6
  of speech   66–7, 71
  of vocal cords   65
Frequency response of hearing aids   133, 136, 167

Fricatives   67, 71
Functional gain   190–1
Fundamental frequency   8

Gain   134, 164–7
  functional   190–1
  insertion   187–90
  open ear   188, 189
Gain control (volume)   82–3
Genetic conditions of the ear   52–3
Genetics   41
German measles   53
Glue ear   48
  see also Otitis media
Grommet   48

Hair cells   28–9, 37
Half gain rule   165
Half peak level (HPL)   196
Half peak level elevation (HPLE)   196
Hard acrylic earmould   178
Harmonic distortion   136–7
Harmonics   8
Head shadow effect   32, 158–9
Hearing aid(s)
  advantages of binaural   157–60
  care and cleaning   210
  evaluation   187–99
  fitting   163–71
  fitting room requirements   163–4
  modification   181–5
  National Health Service   149–52
  practical instruction to
    patients   207–13
  purpose   155
  requirements   155–6
  selection and fitting   155–71
  standards   139–41
  test box   141, 142
Hearing aid components
  amplifier   78–82
  battery   146–9
  microphone   73–8
  output transducer   82
  transistor   78–9
Hearing Aid Council Code of Practice   215–17, 98–101
Hearing aid performance
  frequency response   133, 136, 167
  gain   134
  maximum output   135, 168–70
  specification sheets   132–3

Hearing aid types
  aid conduction   127–32, 156–7
  behind-the-ear   128–9
  bi-CROS   162–3
  bodyworn   127–8
  bone conduction   132, 156–7
  CROS   161
  in-the-canal   130–1
  in-the-ear   130–1
  spectacle   129–30
Hearing loss
  causes, see Medical aspects of
    hearing loss
  in children   253–64
  classification   121–2, 205
  conductive   42–50, 60, 108, 118–
    19, 238, 254–5
  description   121–2
  fluctuating   100
  noise induced   53–4, 98–9
  sensorineural   50–7, 60, 100, 118–
    19
  and speech perception   70–1
  and speech production   71–2, 121
  unilateral   161
Hearing tactics   211–12
Hearing therapist   219–20
Hereditary conditions   42
High frequency emphasis   86–7
  see also Automatic signal processing;
    Venting; Horns
Horns   181, 182
Hydrops, see Menière's disorder

IEC, see International Electrotechnical
    Commission
Impedance
  acoustic   234
  bridge   234–6
Impedance audiometry   232–9
Impression
  of the ear   173
  materials   173–5
  technique   176–8
Incus   25
Induction loop system   213–14
Industrial hearing loss, see Noise
    induced hearing loss
Industrial screening   250
Infection
  inner ear   54–5
  middle ear   47–9

outer ear   44–5
Inner ear
  anatomy   27–30
  congenital conditions   51–3
  pathology   50–7
  physiology   35–9
Innervation of the cochlea   29, 36–9
Input compression   90–1
Insertion gain   145, 166
Insertion gain measurement   187–90
In situ measurement   143–5, 189
Intensity
  sound   6–7
  speech   69–70
Intermodulation distortion   137
Internal noise   138
International Electrotechnical
    Commission   139–40
In-the-canal hearing aid   130–1
In-the-ear hearing aid   130–1
Inverse square law   3, 4, 9
ITE, see In-the-ear hearing aid

KEMAR (Knowles Electronic Manikin
    for Acoustic Research)   144
Kendall toy test   194

Labyrinth   27–8
Labyrinthectomy   58
Libby horn   181
Lip reading   64, 212–13
Localization of sound   32–3
Lombard test   247
Loop system   213–14
Loudness   17
  see also Intensity
Loudspeaker, see Receiver
Low frequency emphasis   86–7

MAF, see Minimum audible field
Malingering deafness   246–7
Malleus   23–5
MAP, see Minimum audible pressure
Maskers, tinnitus   226–7
Masking
  bone conduction   116
  need for   109–10
  noise   115
  procedure   111–13
  rules   110–11
  symbols   114

Mastoid   26
Mastoidectomy   57
Mastoid simulator   145–6
Maximum output   135, 168–70
Maximum power output, *see*
    Maximum output
Meatal projection of earmould   182
Meatus, *see* External auditory meatus
Medical aspects of hearing loss   41–
    60
  inner ear pathology   50–7
  middle ear pathology   46–50
  outer ear pathology   42–6
Medical referral   98–101, 216
Mel, the   17
Ménière's disorder   56
Mercury (mercuric oxide) batteries
    148
Microphone
  capacitor (condenser)   76
  carbon   75
  directional   77–8
  dynamic (moving coil)   75–6
  electret   77
  hearing aid   73–8
  piezo-electric (crystal)   75
  pressure   74
Middle ear
  anatomy   22–7
  function   33
  muscles   34
  pathology   46–50
  physiology   33–5
  transformer action   33, 233–4
Minimum audible field   13, 14
Minimum audible pressure   13
Multichannel hearing aid systems
    91–2, 171
Myringotomy   48, 57

Nasopharynx   30–2
National Health Service hearing aids
    149–52
Nerve supply, *see* Innervation of the
    cochlea
NIHL, *see* Noise induced hearing loss
Noise induced hearing loss   53–4,
    98–9
Noise reduction in hearing aids, *see*
    Automatic signal processing; Bass
    cut; Venting
Non-organic hearing loss   246–9

Occluded ear simulator   142–3
Occlusion effect   35, 108–9
Octave   15
Ohm's Law   85–6
Open ear gain   188, 189
Operations on the ear   57–9
Organ of Corti   28–9
Ossicles   25
Otalgia, *see* Pain in the ear
Otitis externa   45
Otitis media   47–9, 254–5
Otorrhoea, *see* Discharge, ear
Otosclerosis   50
Otoscope   101
Otoscopy   101–3
Ototoxic drugs   55
Outer ear
  anatomy   20–22
  excessive wax   44
  foreign bodies   43
  furunculosis   45
  infection   44–5
  pathology   42–6
  physiology   32–3
  tumours   45–6
Output compression   90, 91
Output limiting   87–92
Output sound pressure level, *see*
    Maximum output
Output transducer   82, 83

Paediatric hearing loss   253–64
Paget's disease   47
Pain in the ear   58–9
Pathology
  inner ear   50–7
  middle ear   46–50
  outer ear   42–6
Patient management, *see*
    Rehabilitation
PB words   192
PC, *see* Peak clipping
Peak clipping   87–8, 170
Perilymph   27
Period   6
Periodic sound   8–9
Phase of sound   7–8
Phon, the   17–18
Phonemes   62, 192
Phonetically balanced (PB) words
    192
Physiology of the ear   32–40

Pink noise   9
Pinna
    anatomy   20–1
    injury to   42–3
    physiology   32
Pitch   17
    see also Frequency
Plosives   67–8, 71
Pre-lingual deafness   253
Presbyacusis   54
Prescription formulae   168
Prescriptive procedures   164–71
Pressure
    audiological reference   11
    minimum audible   7, 13
    sound   6–7
Pseudohypacusis, see Non-organic
    hearing loss
Psychoacoustics   17–18
Psychogenic hearing loss   246
Pure tone audiogram   117
Pure tone audiometry   106–9
Push pull amplifier, see Amplifiers,
    class AB

Radio hearing aid   260–2
Receiver   82, 83
Recommended equivalent threshold
    sound pressure levels   13
Recovery time   139
Recruitment   17
    see also Cochlear hearing loss, tests
    of
Reference coupler   143, 144
Referrable conditions   98–101, 216
Reflex arc   238–9
Rehabilitation
    attitude types   202–3
    practical aspects of   207–13
    process   201–7
    tinnitus   230–2
    see also Hearing aid fitting;
    Subjective evaluation of hearing
    aids
Release time   89, 139
Residual hearing   126
Resistance, electrical   84–5
RETSPL, see Recommended
    equivalent threshold sound
    pressure levels
Reverberation   10
Reverberation time for audiometric

rooms   123
Rinne test   104–5
Rise time   16–17
Room requirements
    for audiometry   122–3
    for hearing aid fitting   163–4
Rubella   53

Saturation sound pressure level, see
    Maximum output
Semicircular canals   27–8
Sensorineural hearing loss   50–7, 60,
    100, 118–19
Shadow curve   109, 110
Short increment sensitivity index test
    244
Signal processing   86–92
SISI test, see Short increment
    sensitivity index test
Social worker   219
Soft acrylic   179
Sone, the   17–18
Sound
    aperiodic   9
    complex   7
    frequency   5–6
    generation   3
    intensity   6–7
    localization   32–3
    measurement   10–14
    perception   35–8
    periodic   8–9
    pressure   6–7
    psychological properties of   17–18
    speed of   3, 6
    transduction   36–8
    transmission   35–6
    wave   3
    wavelength of   5–6
Sound level meter   14
Specification sheets, hearing aid
    132–4
Spectacle hearing aid   129
Specula sterilization   101
Speech
    audiogram   196
    audiometry   191–7
    frequency   65–7
    intensity   69–70
    perception   70–1
    production   63–4, 71–2
    reading   64–5, 217–18

tests   191, 194–7
   therapy   218–19
Speech and intelligibility   61–72
Speech sounds
   vowels   65–7, 71
   consonants   67–8
Speed of sound   3, 6
Spondees   193
Standing waves   8, 10
Stapedectomy   50, 52, 58
Stapedial reflex, *see* Acoustic reflex
Stapedius   34, 237–8
Stapes   25
Stenger test   248
Sterilization of specula   101
Subjective evaluation of hearing aids
   197–9
Surgical treatment, *see* Operations on
   the ear
Syphilis   53

Tactics for new hearing aid users
   211–12
Teacher of the deaf   220
Telecoil switch   84
Telecoil system   213–14
Temporal integration   17
Temporary threshold shift   54
Tensor tympani   34, 238
Test box, hearing aid   141, 142
Test frequencies, audiometric   15
Tinnitus   100, 225
   assessment   227–30
   and associated hearing problems
      226
   conditions involving   59
   loudness matching   229
   maskers   226, 231
   masking evaluation   229–30
   pitch matching   227–8
   rehabilitation   230–2
   relief   226
Tone controls, hearing aid   86–7
Tone decay, *see* Auditory adaptation
Transient distortion   137–8
Transistor   78–9, 85
Travelling wave theory   35–6
Treacher Collins syndrome   42, 46
Treble cut   86–7
'T' switch   84, 214

TTS, *see* Temporary threshold shift
Tubing modification   181–2
Tuning fork   103
Tuning fork tests   104–5
Turner's syndrome   53
Twin channel systems   92
Tympanic cavity   22–6
Tympanic membrane
   anatomy   23–4
   injury to   43
   physiology   33–4
   see also Otoscopy
Tympanogram   236–7
Tympanometer   235–6
Tympanometry   235–9
Tympanoplasty   57–8

ULL, *see* Uncomfortable loudness
   level
Uncomfortable loudness level   116–
   17, 168–70
Unilateral hearing loss   161
Usher's syndrome   52

Venting   181, 182–4
Vertigo   55–7, 99
Vestibular system, *see* Semicircular
   canals
Vibrotactile levels   120
Viruses   45
Vocal cords   63
Vocal tract   63
Voltage   84–5
Volume, *see* Gain; Intensity; Loudness
Volume control, hearing aid   82–3
Vowels   65–7, 71

Waardenburg's syndrome   53
Warble tone   10
Wavelength of sound   5–6
Wave motion   9–10
Waves
   sound   3, 9–10
   standing   8, 10
Wax, excessive   44, 99, 176
Weber test   104
White noise   9

Zinc air batteries   149

Printed in Great Britain
by Amazon.co.uk, Ltd.,
Marston Gate.